Praise for Elizabeth's n

'the most delicious, delightful read of the summer'
The Times (on *Edith and I: On the Trail of an Edwardian Traveller in Kosovo*)

'interesting and inspiring… lively and conversational'
Church Times (on *The Rubbish-Picker's Wife: An Unlikely Friendship in Kosovo*)

'with spirit and humour… this is unusual travel literature'
The Lady (on *Edith and I*)

'A wonderful writer' Matthew Parris

About the Author

Elizabeth Gowing has been practising yoga for twelve years but is still not a likely yogini. She is too fond of cake and to-do lists, and sometimes falls over on her mat. She has done yoga in a cramped carriage on the Trans-Siberian Railway, on a jetty off the Montenegrin coast, in a Kosovan house fortified against blood feuds and as an ice-breaker with a suspicious landlady in Cuba.

This is her fifth travel book (previous titles are *Travels in Blood and Honey: Becoming a Beekeeper in Kosovo, Edith and I: On the Trail of an Edwardian Traveller in Kosovo, The Rubbish-Picker's Wife: An Unlikely Friendship in Kosovo*, and *The Silver Thread: A Journey through Balkan Craftsmanship*). As a speaker she has travelled to over 180 groups around Britain, and the diversity of the communities she has encountered – and the similarity in the ways in which all are working to find meaningful connections – inspired her to take this yoga tour around Britain.

Elizabeth is co-founder of The Ideas Partnership charity that works in Kosovo, using the power of volunteers to tackle education, environmental and cultural heritage challenges, and to support the Roma, Ashkali and Egyptian communities. In 2016 she was awarded the Mother Teresa Medal for humanitarian work by the President of Kosovo, and in 2017 was named by the British Prime Minister as a Point of Light for volunteering around the world.

She is an Arts Society accredited lecturer and frequent contributor to BBC Radio 4.

UNLIKELY POSITIONS

(IN UNLIKELY PLACES)

A Yoga Journey Around Britain

ELIZABETH GOWING

Bradt

First published in the UK in June 2019 by
Bradt Travel Guides Ltd
31a High Street, Chesham, Bucks, HP5 1BW, England
www.bradtguides.com

Print edition published in the USA by The Globe Pequot Press Inc,
PO Box 480, Guilford, Connecticut 06437-0480

Text copyright © 2019 Elizabeth Gowing
Photographs copyright © individual photographers, see below
Edited by Shelagh Boyd
Cover illustration by James Nunn
Layout and typesetting by Ian Spick
Map by David McCutcheon FBCart.S and Ian Spick
Production managed by Sue Cooper, Bradt & Jellyfish Print Solutions

ISBN: 978 1 78477 640 4

British Library Cataloguing in Publication Data
A catalogue record for this book is available from the British Library
Digital conversion by www.dataworks.co.in
Printed in

Photogra
Elizabeth   axton (CP),
Nottingh   oline Greenslade
(CG), Go   ily Vaughen
Lindland

Thanks and Acknowledgements

One of my most treasured yoga memories is not described in this book. It was a class led for me and fifteen of my favourite women who were spending the weekend together. The yoga teacher invited us to stand, one-legged, in the Tree balance pose. However, instead of each of us managing our own instability and insecurity she suggested a 'Forest of Trees' where we were ranged in a circle, palm to palm. As I wobbled for a moment, as someone else's leg tired, the circle pushed back to steady us.

To everyone – in that circle and beyond – who has steadied me during the writing of this book, I give thanks. To everyone mentioned in the book who allowed me to share their stories I am also extremely grateful. Names have been changed in a few cases to protect people's privacy.

And there are specific thanks to offer too – to Jen Barclay, my agent, and Rachel Fielding and Shelagh Boyd at Bradt, who made me feel there was a team cheering for the manuscript despite the lonely process of getting words onto the screen.

To the others who looked through parts of the manuscript, helped me with references or to see how to make it better. Thank you Bar Wilton, Helen Moat, Ian Bancroft, Joanna Griffin, Katie Parry, Kelsey Heeringa, Laura Taylor, Moira Ashley, Paola Fornari Hanna, Robert Wilton, Stephen Fabes and Suzy Pope.

There were some significant logistical challenges in the travels narrated here, and I am grateful, too, for all the help with these. Thank you to Mary and Alan Packer for all the recharging opportunities their hospitality and help has offered – on yoga adventures in Scotland and at Hangjik, their gorgeous Kosovan guesthouse of rural chic – and beyond. Thank you to the Whetham family, to the Stewarts and to

Lesley and Malcolm in Slough for their hospitality as well, to my parents – for this and much more – and to the Raphaels for the 'magic key' to their house which enabled me to come and go and sleep and drink good tea just when I needed to.

And thank you to those who encouraged me on this journey and helped me navigate the world of yoga – to my very first yoga teacher, Elizabeth Reumont, and to Nathalia Berkowitz who taught me later, as well as to Lucy Greeves for suggestions of 'unlikely' places in the yoga landscape.

And to Rob, my repeated Gratitude Diary entry. Thank you, thank you, thank you.

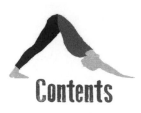

Contents

Chapter 1: Where YouTube Can't Take You 1

Chapter 2: The Village Hall
Port Isaac 10

Chapter 3: Spirit Level
Stand-up Paddleboard Yoga in Nottingham 17

Chapter 4: Balance
On Brimham Rocks, North Yorkshire 23

Chapter 5: Lululemon
Edinburgh.. 30

Chapter 6: Wiped
Hot Yoga and Belonging in Brighton 39

Chapter 7: Doing Time
Yoga in Prison, Surrey.. 48

Chapter 8: Smart Cafés with Mismatched Chairs
Yoga with Asylum Seekers in London 57

Chapter 9: Yoga for People Living with Parkinson's
West Kilbride.. 65

Chapter 10: Upwardly Mobile
Aerial Yoga in Godalming 70

Chapter 11: Downward-facing Doga
Yoga With Your Dog in Shoreditch.............................. 78

Chapter 12: PraiseMoves
A 'Christian Alternative to Yoga' in Peterborough 85

Chapter 13: Kundalini
Awakening the Coiled Serpents of The Cotswolds 99

Chapter 14: Britain's Noisiest City
A Sound Bath in Newcastle 108

Chapter 15: Iyengar Yoga
Maida Vale, London 121

Chapter 16: Yoga Nidra
Stroud 135

Chapter 17: Children's Yoga
Slough 143

Chapter 18: Brahma Kumaris
On the Isle of Man 153

Chapter 19: Pranayama
Liverpool 172

Chapter 20: Laughter Yoga
Blackpool 182

Chapter 21: The Mandala Yoga Ashram
Carmarthenshire 192

Chapter 22: In My End Is My Beginning
Yin Yoga in Newquay 209

Glossary 222

Directory 224

The practitioner will succeed; the non-practitioner will not.
Success in Yoga is not achieved by merely reading books.

Don't indulge in… travel.

The fifteenth-century Hatha Yoga Pradipika manual

A YOGA JOURNEY AROUND BRITAIN

West Kilbride
Yoga for people
with Parkinson's

Edinburgh
Lululemon

Newcastle
Sound Bath

Brimham Rocks
National Trust

Isle of Man
Brahma Kumaris

Blackpool
Laughter Yoga

Liverpool
Pranayama

Nottingham
SUP Yoga

Peterborough
PraiseMoves

Cotswold Wildlife
Park & Gardens

Shoreditch
Doga

Mandala Yoga Ashram
Carmarthenshire

Stroud
Yoga Nidra

Maida Vale
Iyengar Yoga

Hackney City Farm
OURMALA Yoga

Cirencester
Kundalini Yoga

HM Prison Downview

Slough
Children's Yoga

Godalming
Aerial Yoga

Port Isaac
The Village Hall

Brighton
Hot Yoga

Newquay
Yin Yoga

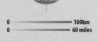

N

Bradt

0 ——————— 100km
0 ——————— 60 miles

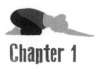

Chapter 1

Where YouTube Can't Take You

'Smith!' screamed the shrewish voice from the telescreen. '6079 Smith W.! Yes, YOU! Bend lower, please! You can do better than that. You're not trying. Lower, please! THAT'S better, comrade.'

I am not a likely yogini: I am too fond of cake and to-do lists. And the start of my yoga journey was a dead end – not just the numbed toes at the ends of my pins-and-needles legs as I cramped my limbs into an unfamiliar half-lotus. There was a sense of futility and frustration in the twists and turns I was forcing myself through.

Perhaps it had been inevitable as I had tried to fast-forward my way to ancient wisdom through 21st-century technology: perhaps it was my fault for trying to learn yoga on YouTube.

The advantages of this approach were seductive – I could fit the yoga sessions in at a time to suit me; no travel time or costs and no need to buy new leggings. No need to worry about what I looked like at all – I could do my practice naked or in my work clothes and no-one would ever see me. It's the greatest gift – perhaps the greatest illusion – offered by the internet to users across the world. No matter if you are poor, maimed, halt or blind… no matter if you are ashamed of what you look like (in general or specifically when squatting in Frog). No matter if you have no skills – whether social skills or the specific skills of *vinyasa* yoga – and no matter if you live far from the corridors of power or the studios of Lululemon; everyone can be connected, the World is Wide open to all through this Web. Find 3G or a Wi-Fi connection and you can be one of us.

So I began with a one-word YouTube search: 'Yoga'…

It yielded an interesting crop of results – some mild pornography, adverts for the 'Yoga' brand laptop which borrows a bit of on-trend Sanskrit as a synonym for flexibility, some Hindi chanting and a wide selection of guided sessions lasting up to an hour. Many advertised themselves like herbalist powders – 'for weight loss', 'for digestion', 'for flexibility', 'for runners', 'for strength', 'for a good night's sleep'. The little capsule-shaped sample window for each one offered to solve every kind of physical, psychic or emotional problem. I could not wait to begin.

The self-diagnosis necessary to select the most appropriate of these sessions for me at any given time was in fact the first benefit that they brought me; often this was the first time I really checked in with myself in a day. The second benefit of e-yoga was being able to have a 'pop-up' approach to my practice. No dimmed lighting, no candles, no preparing of a sacred space. My flat was carpeted so I didn't even lay out a yoga mat. I simply arranged myself cross-legged in the middle of my sitting room and opened a new window on my laptop. And yet, the space did become sacred. It hushed, as I silenced the multiple conversations I conducted sometimes simultaneously on Facebook, on my phone, on Skype. And I silenced the conversations in my head too ('should I do that?' 'why did I say that?' 'why did she say that?' 'am I good enough?' 'am I fat?' 'am I happy?' 'was that right?'). With a click I was focused on somewhere else.

Incongruously, I could feel that I was living by the precepts of the fifteenth-century Hatha Yoga Pradipika manual – 'Yoga succeeds by these six: enthusiasm, openness, courage, knowledge of the truth, determination, and solitude.'

It was a solitude which still allowed me to inhale and exhale in time with the group of girls in black Lycra filmed doing their sequences by a Joshua tree in the desert; for a while I had a regular date with a guy in his garage. I watched only once the three women who squabble over whose turn it is to give instruction, but worked through a series of cat-like women demonstrating each pose in their sequences with fluid grace, before unwinding and bitchily saying 'if that's a little challenging for you then look at Suzy here' gesturing to a dumpier model off to one side and demonstrating how the pose can be made possible for a normal body.

Once I had got into a routine of regular sessions 'on the mat' – or at least on the trackpad – I made sure that if I was going to be somewhere without internet access I used a DVD a friend had lent me. This 'enlightenment to go' had been a rather surprising McDonald's free gift, and its production values were those of a Happy Meal. As many yogis had been involved in the filming as strawberries had been required for the flavoured milkshakes – this was a yoga session which took place entirely within a CGI lab. It featured a tight-abbed model with a fixed serene smile reminiscent of the women by the Joshua tree. She moved with the dreamy glide of a video-game character in a way that was more a reminder of the complete absence of friction in her world than a motivation to yogic discipline.

But I realised that the experience of following the practice of the yogis and yoginis who peopled the other sessions I watched on screen wasn't so different from mimicking this automaton. I was removed from the physical experience of their body heat and sweat by the camera and screen which divided us. And their lives moved on different planes from mine: what was a brief spontaneous hour for them became a repeated, rewound and paused reality for me. I was shocked to find that one of the teachers leading a session had, when I found her in another online video, aged and become pregnant. How was that possible when I'd seen her only yesterday all young and slim-waisted?

There were some parts of their lives I knew far better than them; perhaps they had rehearsed their recorded sessions once or twice but they couldn't have watched them as many times as I had. And in many cases it didn't seem that they had cared very much about their production values, based on nothing more than a GoPro camera and a quiet Sunday morning. In one session filmed in Adriene's sitting room, her large dog enters from behind the camera. Padding up to her affectionately despite the fact that she is – and therefore I am too – in a yogic squat, he licks her face as she hovers in the preparation pose for Crow. With lactic acid screaming in my thighs I railed at this slobbery delaying tactic each time I ran the video.

A different yoga teacher set up his camera on a boardwalk over a lake. It was set in a quiet park and a tranquil background for our Sun Salutation series, but it wasn't a private space, and as Tim athletically jumped to Plank pose or lowered himself in the half press-up of Chaturanga there were curious observers behind him. Some stood and stared, and though Tim was oblivious, the viewers at home could see it, and I found myself oddly conflicted. Because we, too, were voyeurs of Tim's practice, but at the same time the curious faces which peered ever closer over his shoulder and into the lens of the camera were not just staring at a camera: they were looking right into our eyes. And I was in my front room, not wearing very much, and I didn't want to be stared at like that.

Of course, any connection with these teachers was an illusion but it was a powerful one that the teachers encouraged. They greeted me at the beginning of the recording, and they said things like 'well done; that's beautiful' while I was holding the poses. *How did they know?* At that point I could have popped out of the room. But I didn't. And part of the reason was that there was someone there talking to me: 'Smith!' screamed the shrewish voice from the telescreen. '6079 Smith W.! Yes, YOU! Bend lower, please! You can do better than that. You're not trying. Lower, please! THAT'S better, comrade.'

Sometimes I felt like it was 1984 again.

In fact the real events of the year 1984 had included my first experience of yoga, through a book belonging to my mother. The cover showed a woman with long loose hair and a leotard, and the text inside told me why I should eat fresh vegetables (spices will 'destroy the life-force value of many foods') and elevate my feet whenever possible. The night after I first found the book, I had unscrewed the legs at the head of my bed so that I could sleep with my feet higher than my head. I woke up the next morning with my chest uncomfortably compressed, and from then until finding yoga available online had not experimented further with it (and not much more with fresh vegetables).

Decades passed and one morning I was stretching out in bed and idly played with lifting a leg up above my head. That's where I knew the leg was going, where I knew it could go but… I was unsettled to discover that it could in fact no longer get there. I wasn't unfit – I'd run a half marathon just a few months earlier – but I was disconcertingly inflexible. This happened in December, just as I was preparing for my usual serious round of New Year resolutions. I remembered then the leotard lady in my mother's book. The text had said that:

> People who undertake to perform the Yoga exercises…
> stimulate the 'Life-Force' almost immediately. The body
> begins to recondition itself, producing all of the wonderful
> results which I know you want… START YOUR YOGA
> EXERCISES… NOW.

It was in capitals! So I had resolved that when January came around I would START.

The exercises were not easy, and the new language I learned was not just verbs. The teachers' instructions were spiced with Sanskrit so I learned to control my *drishti* – my gaze, focusing on a particular point. I became acquainted with a menagerie of animals, and some of their names in Sanskrit too – dogs ('upward-facing', 'downward-facing' and 'puppy'), the butterfly, the camel, the cat, the cow (and the 'face of a cow'), the cobra, dolphin, fish, frog, pigeon, crow and eagle. My yoga workshop also included some practical equipment – bridge, boat, bow, chair, plank and plough – and some new mentors: the cobbler, the dancer, the hero, the warrior.

So this was the motley crew who accompanied me on my new online yoga journey. The impact on my life was rather hit and miss, though I was able to find some patterns in the habits of mind and approach shared by the YouTube people who'd made yoga part of their life. I stopped going for the occasional massages that had been a favourite indulgence – I found that a good yoga session gave me far more of the sensation of being liquid-limbed, and was also cheaper. On a good day I got glimpses of mind-body-spirit connection that took me beyond mere 'stretchiness in Sanskrit'. I set an intention for the class, holding someone or some aspiration, some pattern of thought, in the forefront of my focus and honouring it with each breath. I lay in *Shavasana* at the end of the practice and was able to take my mind away from particular twinges of muscle or mind, to hover above my dear, flawed, perfect little body lying on the floor and to see that it was in fact lying on the surface of the earth and that the earth was spinning through space. I recognised that my breath and my consciousness formed a marvellous flickering flame for me to nurture, and that the breath and consciousness of others were born from the same fire and to be nurtured. Sometimes these epiphanies stayed with me as limbs creaked me off the carpet and into the realities of life where baggage literally and metaphorically tugged at my carefully realigned shoulders.

From these sessions I also started to develop an instinct for what was useful yoga practice, either physically or psychologically, and what was cynical snake-oil salesmanship. When one day I watched a 'Yoga Meltdown' session I should have realised just from the name that this was unlikely to be staying true to the principles of yoga I'd started to isolate as inspiring and useful. The session leader announced that she'd be taking some yoga moves and 'pumping them up'. When I heard her tell us to 'melt your arms down' before adding, almost in satire, 'that's yoga speak for stretching as far as you can go' (which it isn't, actually) my indignation told me that I had identified something in yoga practice that meant enough to me that I was willing to defend it, even if only by muttering at a computer screen.

At the end of the online classes the teachers would say '*namaste*' and I would whisper 'namaste' self-consciously back in my silent room. Before the video ended the teachers would add hopefully 'do leave your comments on our fan page' and sometimes I even found myself reading these, eager to make contact with others teetering on the same path to enlightenment as me. Adriene has built a legendary online yoga community, with weekly newsletters written in her Girl Next Door style that you can't help but find likeable.

'I am committed to doing everything in my power to make [home practice] feel easier instead of more difficult, authentic instead of false, and connected versus shallow', she said in an email that came right into my inbox, addressed 'Hello Elizabeth'. And 'I keep knocking on your door to see if you can play'. I was developing a bit of a pash for Adriene, like you might have for one of those talented sixth-formers you can watch from across the school hall, but to whom you can't ever speak.

Eventually, however, for all the talk of community, I realised that smileys couldn't replace a real smile, or emoticons replace emotions. If I really cared about those flickers of consciousness in others and if I wanted a sense of real community I needed to try yoga with people occupying at least three dimensions. I needed to enrol in a class.

A class would give me a better understanding of yoga 'on the mat'. I'd get feedback on how I was holding myself and I'd be able to share my journey with other people in real time. But I also felt a hunger for understanding how yoga took you off the mat; to hear from real people about the ways it changed their behaviour, their relationships, their health and happiness. What if my journey could be both internal and external? I had heard of yoga being offered in Britain's hot spots and beauty spots, read claims of it building communities of refugees, building bodies of people living with disabling illness, building peace for people in prison. I knew there was children's yoga, yoga for dogs, yoga of the breath, yoga of the mind, yoga of sound, karma yoga of service to others, and laughter yoga. My tongue did yoga positions of its own, learning new names for yoga approaches like Iyengar, Kundalini, or Yin. With all these stretches and twists going on around Britain I wondered what I could learn about my country from watching them in action; and what I could learn about myself.

But first things first: before I could find out how yoga could reveal the rest of modern Britain to me, I needed to learn what it could teach me about my home. I headed down to the village hall.

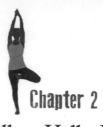

Chapter 2

The Village Hall – Port Isaac

'Set an intention'

'Set an intention for the class.' Tracey had a singsong voice and a serene dolphin smile which she directed at each of us in turn as she looked around the hall in our small seaside village.

She invited us to scan our bodies, 'not judging, just noticing'. I was familiar with this from my online classes. One teacher had suggested imagining a beam of light cascading over your body from above. Another had made it more tangible – 'break an egg over your skull and let it drip down every contour of your body.'

'Now come to a comfortable seated position at the top of your mat.' There was a cracking as the group folded their knees into place. It was like snapping driftwood for kindling.

Even though I was the youngest here by twenty years I was the last into position, distracted by Tracey's previous instruction. An *intention*? What was it that I was *intending* to happen here? In fact, why was I here?

I was here for the same reason I had been at the village Heritage Centre committee meeting last week, even though my attempts there were scuppered by me making a clumsy joke about the local sea-shanty group, The Fisherman's Friends, which I felt had gone down badly with the wife of a shanty-singer.

I was here today for the same reason I'd started using nautical vocabulary like 'scuppered'. I was carefully weaving into my conversation local phrases wherever I could; even though I still had upcountry ways, at least I now knew to call it *upcountry*.

Tracey caught my eye. 'Trikonasana,' she repeated, and I looked around to catch a belated cue from the spry ladies stretching on either side of me.

'Hold on to your intention,' she reminded us and a wobble passed through the room as we yoginis tried to hold the pose at the same time as remembering something from ten minutes before. I lost my concentration on the poses again.

Why was I here? Not just in this village hall today but why had we come to make a home in this small Cornish village at all? I was allergic to lobster, which was the only thing the fishermen could make money from here now. And I didn't yet have views on parking, rubbish collection or planning permission, which seemed to be how to make conversation in the shops.

There was an irony in the fact that it had been Cornwall's wild isolation which had attracted us here – big skies, and beaches marked only by the footprints of seabirds. Perched on the cliff, our new home was to be a garret from which we'd write rolling prose to the sound of the waves. We'd go for a daily run along the coastal path and then we'd sup on ice cream. We had been wearied by commuter crowds crashing like surf around London Underground ticket gates in the morning and we had moved here in search of the simplicity of empty spaces and a community where you would look people in the eye when you passed them in the street, and you might find that you could then hail them by name.

This morning I'd found the emptiness of a sparse yoga class of strangers in a village hall. Was I really trying to fit in here? A woman in middle age standing in Tree pose in a forest of retirees on the far western edge of Britain?

'Focus on your breath,' Tracey prompted gently and I tried to bring my focus into the things I could control.

There was a noise outside the hall, and Tracey lost concentration as well:

'Oh gosh, it's recycling day today and I forgot to put my bin out,' she said. Yes, unlike those asynchronous, anonymous YouTube teachers, this class was being led in real time. It was recycling day for me too, and I had also forgotten to put my bin out. From the look of panic on the face of the woman next to me – whom I was calling Hilda, though I later discovered that it was not her name – she had forgotten as well. I felt a sudden, pleasing surge of connection with the bodies in this room and the shared life that we and our separated waste were living.

I was working hard at connections. I had made myself start a Gratitude Diary, having read about the 'thnx4.org' initiative at the University of California, which invited people to keep anonymised online journals which were then analysed, together with the impact of gratitude practices on their mental health and happiness, as assessed in online tests. In fact I had tired of going online to post what I was grateful for, but was hooked on the habit of forcing myself to notice. I was now writing down every morning the first new thing I was grateful for (*first* because I wanted to start the day looking out for the good stuff; *new* because otherwise, most mornings I found I would write nothing more than the extreme good fortune I have in the man I wake up next to).

And now I was practising sharing gratitude so that I passed on my thanks, wrote to companies, sent messages to the friends who had been responsible for whatever I'd been grateful for. The owner of a Port Isaac gift shop where I'd bought a ring, and noted it in the gratitude diary, one day got an email telling her how I appreciated it. She wrote me a kind message back and I felt the skein of gratitude meshing together the fishing village. Along with the yoga I was consciously and carefully trying to gather other tools to make sense of my new life here.

On one leg in front of us Tracey was teaching us to hold the balance pose and extend it with each of our exhalations. It was this link between movement and the breath that in my eclectic online experiences had come to define yoga. In the stillness of the room, we could hear the sea outside, breathing in and out like the shingly rasp of 'Hilda' next to me.

Tracey took us into a Sun Salutation series, even as the weather outside was fit to obliterate any sun. She used the Sanskrit names for the poses and as I strained into uncomfortable half push-ups, my mind enjoyed the gymnastics it was more adept at, spotting patterns in the language; parsing the syllables with fluency even while my muscles throbbed and failed at the positions the words described. I'd tried this way into Cornwall too, enrolling in Cornish evening classes at the local secondary school; I could understand the place names now – the *tre*, *pol* and *pen* 'by which ye may know all Cornishmen'; the *lan* sacred enclosures and the *wheals* that don't turn, except in the workings of the mines they recall; the fact that in 'Redruth' one syllable means 'red' but it's the second one. *Red* in Cornish means 'ford'. But I had no-one to try out my new language with – except my enthusiastically inconsistent language teacher. In the first depressing lesson he had explained that the last surviving Cornish first-language speaker died in the eighteenth century.

Next came the Warrior series. Warrior I has you lunging forward, knee never quite bent to the ninety degrees you're bidden to, and arms up in the air as you look up. It feels more reverent than martial. But then you move into Warrior II which is one of my favourite poses – the legs held in the same position but the arms stretched out, one in front and one behind. You can look out along them – to check alignment but also to note your body's musculature, staring at it for longer than would be considered seemly in any other context. Then there's Warrior III, a balancing pose on one leg; the other stretched out at ninety degrees behind you and the arms following the line of the leg, stretched straight in front. One YouTube teacher had called the pose 'Superman'.

And finally, a delicious stretch after the muscles strained in the preceding three, there was Peaceful Warrior where the legs were back on the ground but the arms windmilled so that the back hand lay along its corresponding leg and the other hand reached to the sky.

'Now come down gently onto your mats,' Tracey directed us, 'and lie on your backs.'

She took us through stretches like bringing the knees into the chest – which always seems designed for people without breasts. The thought occurred to me that it might even have been designed by *men*. We twisted and we folded, lying our torsos on top of our thighs with stomach, as Claire Dederer describes it, 'curled like a fat little dog onto your lap'.

'We're coming to the end of our practice and it's time for Shavasana, the final relaxation.' There was a murmur of anticipation about Corpse pose that the pensioners hadn't shown for any of the other positions we'd worked through.

'Get a blanket if you've brought one,' Tracey advised. Hilda had brought a duvet with her, and tucked it up under her chin, before obediently closing her eyes and letting her jaw go slack. She reminded me of Grandma Josephine in *Charlie and the Chocolate Factory*.

Tracey was taking us through a guided relaxation.

'Remember your intention,' she said.

I remembered – I was wanting to work out why I was here and how I was going to fit in. How could I stay true to me and still find some point of connection here? I lay on my mat, feeling the meat of me settle around the restlessness of what Tracey called the 'monkey mind'. She was walking slowly round the room now and as she passed me she caught my eye and smiled at me. And I realised I didn't need to *work out*. I didn't need to set my monkey off on the puzzle of how to fit in – being here was enough, with these women who had smiled and spoken to me just because I was present.

I let my gaze wander round the hall – at the sign which said that the hall had been redecorated by local boy Laurence Llewelyn-Bowen; at the other bodies which peopled this space where I lived, and which I was now getting to know. There had been a time that everyone in this village would have known one another through birth or marriage; women would have worked the pilchard catch together. Now there was a village Facebook group but with most of the local shops turned into holiday homes to serve visiting tourists, there were not many options for women to come together and grunt in unison. The church was one, the pub was another, and soon becoming my favourite was this village hall.

At the end of the time in Shavasana, to close the class, Tracey said a gentle 'namaste' with her hands held at her chest, palms facing, like a child's prayer.

'It means "the divine light in me salutes the divine light in you,"' she explained. There was a murmuring reply of 'namaste' from everyone on their mats, and I said it too, self-consciously. I imagined the divine light rather like the pilot light in the boiler we'd had to buy for our old London flat (though not something available to us in this part of Cornwall: no gas mains round here). And if I had that tremulous blue blaze within me then so did Tracey (it was readily visible and I easily saluted it) and Hilda and the rest. We rolled up our mats together, grimacing at the protesting muscles we had in common, preparing to walk home, limber-limbed through the village's lanes. I imagined us as if in a memorial procession each holding these tiny flames – perhaps like the women of the village would have done in the time of the nighttime pilchard catch as they navigated by lantern through the dark, spotting the swaying lights of their neighbours and making answering call.

Gratitude diary entry:
waking to Rob's breathing

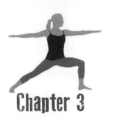

Chapter 3

Spirit Level – Stand-up Paddleboard Yoga in Nottingham

'Every action has a reaction'

The sea is an active member of the Port Isaac community, like an elderly relative always sat in the corner and whose moods of anger or placidity set the tone for the day. It's a business partner for fishermen and the tourist trade; it's an artist's model and it's a playmate. Never had I thought it could be a yoga teacher.

But then I read about stand-up paddleboard, or SUP, yoga. The idea seemed absurd – I had enough difficulty balancing in some poses when I was held up by the splintery solidity of the village hall floorboards. And I had never even Stood Up on a Paddleboard, let alone lunged on one or waged Warrior on it.

Added to this, I have a difficult relationship with watersports. I love the sea and am a competent if unenthusiastic swimmer, but when I went in a canoe as a child I had a frightening experience combining the panic of claustrophobia with the trauma of public failure and social embarrassment. I was probably eight at the time and had gone out on the water with the sons of family friends who were older and far more capable than me. I couldn't follow their instructions, set my small craft lurching with every attempt to get moving, and then tried vainly – and dangerously – to get out of the canoe, which only set them shouting at me more, their voices bouncing with a distorted jeer off the water's surface. As I struggled further, the voices were joined by those of our parents watching from the shore (possibly only a few metres away, but in my memory too, too far), and a private incompetence seemed to be rapidly transforming into public humiliation.

With one exception – a whim when on my own by a glassy and isolated lake in Canada as an adult – I hadn't taken anything smaller than a boat out on the water since. No surfboards, no kayaks, and certainly nothing as unforgiving as a stand-up paddleboard.

I explained this to Cassie as we stood on the edge of a lake in Nottingham. She seemed unbothered at having at her side a rookie seeking closure for their experience of childhood distress. 'You'll be fine!' she said breezily. 'Really, you will.'

Why is it that we trust some people instinctively? In wobbly moments over the next hour the thought did occur to me that I knew nothing about Cassie's credentials, though I later read about her Yoga Alliance and RNLI lifesaving qualifications. But she'd said I'd be fine. And I was. She'd said I'd be fine. *So* I was.

I wondered whether it was related to us being similar. Similar age, similar build. This was a bit like having a dialogue with my better self.

It was also definitely helped by the fact that, despite my visions of attempting Dancer pose while being rocked by waves, my session with Cassie took place on a lake of reassuringly still waters in Nottingham.

It wasn't my first visit to Nottingham, but reflecting on my previous visits – for National College of School Leadership training, and a christening – I worried that this would turn out to be a dangerous mixture of the two. I really didn't want to be baptised today. Cassie's instructions ahead of the class had inspired confidence ('you won't need to wear a wetsuit; wear your regular fitness gear') but still left room for a fear that dragged at me like wet clothes ('bring a change of outfit, just in case').

'You seem nervous,' my taxi driver had said as we drove from the station to the lake, and I'd had to admit that he was right. I explained what I was travelling to the lake for and he was interested to learn about yoga. 'This is a good city,' he said. 'You learn about other religions here, not just in theory but in practice.' He had been born in Nottingham but had then moved to Heathrow to work at the airport. He'd come back home because he liked it here – 'a peaceful city,' as he said. But now he was on the verge of another move, with the possibility of going back to London where a friend was offering the opportunity for him to work as a cab driver with better pay. But to do that he'd have to leave his wife and his kids, aged ten and eight, while he set up their new life in the capital. 'Every action has a reaction,' he said wisely. 'And what might seem like the best thing to do for my family's future might bring about a reaction that makes things worse for them now.'

The philosophy ran in my head – and rippled around my feet – as I took my first unsteady step onto the paddleboard. The board looked flimsy in the water – more like a piece of toast kept afloat by chance before the ducks got it than a plinth which I could inhabit and move around on for the next hour. Cassie showed me how to ease onto it, holding my centre of gravity low. I got onto it on my knees and shuffled into place, keeping the middle of my body over the stripe down the middle of the board, and the paddleboard's handle under my tummy button as I'd been told. Each shuffle brought a lurch from the board and the feeling of a surge below me; every action a reaction.

I stopped to take stock… which was a bad thing to do because the point at which I stopped was a point at which my middle was not over the middle of the board. Everything tilted, and with a wave of pondweed smell (*weed*, like the past tense of 'to urinate') memories came into focus of that Welsh waterside more than thirty years before.

But today I had Cassie. She didn't shout at me and she didn't laugh at me, and eventually we got an anchor weighed to hold the board fast, and got me lying down on my back on the board. That was not before I had got my feet wet in a slosh of water that came onto the paddleboard. Despite the water's surprisingly silken touch on my toes, never had the Shavasana position seemed so hard-won.

Cassie told me we would start with some relaxation.

'So first check whether you're storing any tension,' she said, and instead of releasing, the muscles of my face twitched into an involuntary smile.

Tension? Of course I'm storing flipping tension! I'm trying to keep dry on a tiny bit of Styrofoam in the middle of a lake. I'm trying to face down childhood demons even though they're sneaking up on me to tug me into the deeps with every shift of my body.

Nevertheless, I tried to scan my body, to let go (but not of that magic line drawn on the board to which I had to keep symmetrical). My board drifted under a willow tree so that light came to me dappled, and occasionally a leaf tickled my face while I lay like Ophelia, thinking about 'muddy death'. I had looked at an information board near the lake before the class started, and the list of plants I could get tangled up in made for great Anglo-Saxon poetry. *Bogbean, lesser water parsnip, water dropwort, fool's watercress, spike-rush, common club-rush*… I called myself all of these things and worse for attempting to negotiate with water when we had come to such a definite stand-off more than three decades ago. Round my ankle was a Velcro cuff attached to a long tough leash, so I wouldn't lose the board even if I fell in. It made me feel like Princess Leia with the water as Jabba. I was aware of feeling enslaved, and not in a good way.

Cassie's voice floated around me – she was steering her own board to keep up with the wandering course of mine – as she talked me through deep breathing. Her words got distorted off the water and the end of her sentences came from a different direction from where she'd started speaking. It was how I imagined the voice of God might sound – giving reassuring instructions from everywhere and nowhere. I could feel myself starting to settle. Perhaps I wasn't going to drown today. Perhaps I wouldn't even make a fool (or a bogbean) of myself.

My mind was wandering and I focused as Cassie directed me gently but firmly into a Tabletop position. This was the first time I had ever been in a yoga class one-to-one, and I realised there was nowhere to hide. When the lady on YouTube said 'pull your abdominal muscles in' it was a remote suggestion recorded by someone who might be on the other side of the globe, and whom I would never meet. Frankly, I could push my tummy out, go and make a cup of tea, or just switch her to silent if I wanted. In the village hall when Tracey had told us to pull in our abdominals, she had cast her eye around the group, and as a teacher myself used to thirty primary school pupils I knew she could, and would, note any obvious rebels or stragglers, but the precise position of an individual's abdominals was really for them to decide. Here there was no escape. 'No, pull them in more than that,' came the disembodied voice across the water. 'That's it!' She was watching me.

And even if she hadn't been, there was an even more attentive teacher just waiting to ripple me over the knuckles if I didn't hold my Tabletop pose symmetrically; the irrefutable feedback of the lake's meniscus told me immediately if I wasn't keeping straight. My SUP had become an enormous spirit level.

Shavasana had seemed like a triumph, but to hold Tabletop pose was true victory. This was pretty much officially a yoga position.

And I was doing it on the water! Cassie saw my back straightening in satisfaction.

'Oh, we'll get you doing more than that,' she promised, and talked me through the movements into a pose she called Wild Thing, and then into the beginnings of Bridge pose. 'Just be careful,' she warned with the slightest of tremors in her voice. 'I did once have a woman in class who went into Bridge pose and then up into a shoulder stand and back into Plough… and off the end of the board.'

Despite the tremor I managed an adapted Side Plank (bottom leg bent under me for support), an adapted Triangle pose (again, with the back leg kneeling on the board), and a Warrior series with my back leg still anchoring me.

In between, I even freed up some mental space to be able to talk to Cassie. She said that she did also teach what she called 'matted yoga'; the word and the way she used it made it sound clotted and tangled in comparison with what we were doing today; it made me feel combed out and free. And she said she'd experimented with other approaches to yoga too, leading naked yoga classes and yoga in nearby caves. Suddenly what I was doing with her here today seemed really quite straightforward.

Finally, she got me up on my feet, and with pride and poise I held a standing Warrior pose above the swirling green of the lake. I looked out along the fleshy waves around the muscle and bone of my forward arm, and felt my drishti focus piercingly on a waterside in 1981. I looked it full in the eye, and then very gently withdrew my gaze and my arms, and Cassie talked me through paddling the board back to shore.

Gratitude diary entry
chocolate cantucci biscuits given to me by a friend

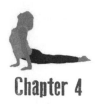

Chapter 4

Balance – on Brimham Rocks, North Yorkshire

'Shall we turn that down? It's not very mindful, is it'

'Where Yorkshire grit meets mindfulness', the publicity material promised, so I reserved my place on the yoga class to be held at the National Trust's property at Brimham Rocks. The rock formations are made up of towering boulders – most of them rounded, to add to their implausibility – stacked like Zen pebbles or massive Andy Goldsworthy sculptures. Newly enthused by having conquered the wobbles in Nottingham I felt that this would be an extraordinary place to practise balance.

To be there on time, my rucksack and I needed to spend the previous night in Harrogate. As usual, I looked for the cheapest place I could find on Airbnb, and I found a 'superhost' called Charlie offering a great price and glowing reviews.

Charlie welcomed me and asked about breakfast.

'I guess it will be vegetarian?'

I smiled. 'Yes, but how did you know?'

'Oh, doing this you become expert at getting to know people. I spotted a vegan once.'

Like all his reviews had promised, Charlie was keen to give his local knowledge, but when he heard that I was going to Brimham Rocks in the morning he grimaced. 'That's where all the teenagers go to smoke pot.' Perhaps he saw my face fall; 'But at least you've got nice weather forecast,' he added, looking on the bright side. Really?

It seemed unlikely – I'd just got back from a hot southeast European summer and England was feeling chilly. I checked online: a dry day with a low of six degrees centigrade and a high of sixteen. I shivered.

I was in touch with some local friends, Su and Paddy, too. I mentioned that I was wary about having too much time to hang around at the site outside if the temperatures were going to be so unfriendly. Su's response was, 'Ha! BTW sixteen degrees is summer up here.' She said she'd be taking sun cream out with her tomorrow, but I reminded myself that this was a cold county, unused to good weather – Yorkshire has nineteen per cent more rain than the UK average.

The next morning, once I'd bought some leggings at Primark, my taxi drove me the twenty minutes to the moor through what I had to admit was a bright day, past dry-stone walls and gorse and bluebells to get to the National Trust land. I knew we'd arrived when I saw a wooden (biodegradable) plaque in the distinctive National Trust font. The carefully carved sign announced 'ice cream van parking; please keep clear'. This was a parking lot that had its priorities right.

From here I could walk up through the eerie landscape of balancing rock formations as high as houses. Often the stones at the top were larger than those which supported them and it seemed like they could fall at any moment, though they had apparently been around for 320 million years. You didn't need to smoke pot here.

The site was still relatively empty, with the landscape filled only with a few families exploring, and the occasional shapes of National Trust staff with their distinctive bouncy walk and the shorts they seem to wear whatever the weather.

Since I was early I went in to the visitor centre to leave my rucksack and to look around. Inside there was a 'web' for visitors to 'weave' their impressions into, with slips of paper that could be twined as weft into the woollen warp. There was no-one else in the room but the slips of paper were a way of sharing this view with others; as if there were fellow voices murmuring 'dramatic', 'calm', 'natural beauty', 'serene', 'makes me want to climb' and the perhaps obvious but certainly accurate 'rocks! rocks! rocks!'.

The yoga class was being run as part of the site's 'Mindful May' promotion and downstairs in the shop I saw more mindfulness (commercial?) opportunities like their *Colouring for Mindfulness; Art Therapy to Help You Unwind* book with designs based on the rock formations.

The shop was quiet with just one member of staff, at the till, and we were interrupted only by her walkie-talkie exploding occasionally into an uncomfortably loud crackle and whine that made us both wince.

'Shall we turn that down?' she said eventually. 'It's not very mindful, is it.' It was a fair point, and the first sign that Mindful May might be more than a publicity gimmick. Perhaps this month really would leave the place – the world – with a bit less deafening chatter.

I didn't buy a colouring book, or even some mindless local Harrogate toffee. I scanned the shelves remembering what the Pradipika had to say about diet:

> These are wholesome for the best yogis: wheat, rice, barley, shashtika rice, ... milk, ghee, sugar, butter, sugar candy, honey, dry ginger, cucumbers, the five potherbs, mung dahl etc. and pure water.

It seemed that Kendal mint cake might just about qualify, and anyway that's what I felt one should buy at a National Trust site. Once

I had it I was equipped for a long hike but instead I just wandered slowly outside because Charlie had been right; this was a beautiful day and it was no hardship to sit and wait for the class in the early summer sunshine.

There were huge old boulders by the drinks kiosk, blotted with lichen that made them look like ancient scarred whales. I leant against one, drinking some Harrogate spa water and feeling dwarfed by nature. The day was clear enough to be able to see even beyond the rock formations, across the forty miles to the nearby power station, as if the yoga class had started already. I was being offered images of balance, clarity and might.

Soon it really was time to start and ten of us who'd gathered were led by our teacher, Caroline, to a secluded space within the site. She acknowledged that some of the group might be new to yoga, as well as attracted by the opportunity for a no-commitment taster in a special setting, and she guided us as we quietly colonised the space with multicoloured sticky mats.

We started with some meditation, with Caroline telling us to sit up 'whether cross-legged or kneeling, but in a position that's comfortable and dignified, as if we're about to do something special – because we are'. It was a beautiful place to meditate; a beautiful place just to be. We were focused for a while on our breathing, and I took in the smell of summer with each inhalation. There was cut grass and soft warm breeze.

'In…hale,' said Caroline with a pause between syllables that made me think of *hale* as in hearty.

'Ex…hale,' she followed, and this time I heard the syllable like a greeting to Caesar. *All hail!*

My mind was wandering.

I was wondering whether I should have shopped around more before buying those leggings; they were cutting into me uncomfortably. Then I thought of the woman in the visitor centre shop and gently I said to myself, 'Shall we turn that down? It's not very mindful, is it.' Obediently, the trivial thoughts floated away. Of course it wasn't long before new thoughts came – just as trivial – but I tried the technique again, hushing my internal walkie-talkie.

After our period of silent breathing, Caroline read us the poem called 'The Peace of Wild Things' by Wendell Berry, and when the meditation was over we could open our eyes to feast as he had on the view. Here we were looking straight over to the Menwith Hill listening station, squat and strange in the landscape like a metaphor. But otherwise our view had nothing manmade in it and as we started the physical part of our practice it was exhilarating to be able to stretch your hand up in a Triangle pose and be reaching for the sky (as Wendell Berry would have it, 'I feel above me the day-blind stars waiting with their light'); when we were in Mountain pose we really were rooted directly to the ground, not through laminate flooring and reinforced concrete. When we came down to our mats, we inhaled the scent of fresh earth lightly peppered with fresh sweat.

Caroline said that she had taken the opportunity to teach yoga in this special space because of this power of taking your practice outside so that yoga can reconnect you both to your body and to the earth. She scanned our group – heterogeneous in age and body type – and clearly made a guess at the demographics, based on who-knows-what instincts and intersections of auras, National Trust membership and geography.

'You might be stiff,' she said. It was always true, and my yoga teachers had often mentioned it, usually in the context of the time spent bent over laptops or other electronic devices. But Caroline's assessment was different. 'Perhaps you've been gardening,' she hazarded. That was the point when I knew I was at a National Trust yoga session.

To loosen up our stiffness – even for those of us who had done no gardening in years – she led us through an Earth sequence with Dru Yoga influences that was new to me. Standing tall with hands hanging loose, we interlinked our cupped fingers and then used them to 'raise the energy' up from the earth, as if we were scooping water from a river and lifting the hands up to our heart. Then turning the hands over so that the palms now faced the ground, the movement went in reverse until the arms were straight down, at which point the motion continued with the palms pushing outwards and the arms lifting upwards again, past chest-height and on to being held up above the head. Then we released our hands and stretched fingers wide out to the side, as if we could encompass all this landscape, all this beauty, and gather it to us. We repeated until the movement had become, as they say, 'second nature', though that presupposes what 'first nature' might be.

As we worked I started to feel stinging along my shoulders – Su had been wiser than I had about how the day would heat up. I was stupid for not having brought sun cream, but at the same time it reinforced my connection here with the elements. In my outdoor yoga practice not only had I 'saluted' the sun but the sun had saluted me.

The session closed with some 'floor work' though here our *floor* was dandelions. When Caroline told us to 'open like a flower' it felt not just like a simile, but a way of encouraging us to attend to an instruction manual studded all around us in the landscape. Thinking about the flora here made me realise the absence – with the notable exception of the Lotus pose – of flowers in yoga: the session here was not only taking yoga to the Yorkshire landscape, but bringing this rich landscape into yoga.

I remembered the bluebells I'd seen tingeing the verges on the way here, the marzipan of gorse flowers, the bishop-purple bubbles of bell heather flowers on the moor's Site of Special Scientific Interest. I focused on these images of fragility in tough conditions: they were vivid symbols of what it can look like when 'Yorkshire grit meets mindfulness', and what you gain from sharpening your focus. When I rolled up my mat and began my journey home through the improbable rocks, I resolved to do more walkie and less talkie.

Gratitude diary entry
the softness of a fleecy bath mat underfoot in the bathroom of my Airbnb

Chapter 5

Lululemon – Edinburgh

'The humanist ideal of unconditional positive regard'

Sunday morning in Edinburgh, and it was definitely the morning after. I arrived on the night bus and wandered blearily through the streets looking for somewhere to recharge (myself, my computer) before my 'Hair of the Down Dog' yoga class at the Lululemon studio. Few places were open and the café where I finally came to rest had menus on every table with the slogan 'DRINK DRANK DRUNK'.

I didn't really need breakfast so much as a bed to curl up in, but the menus also offered the next best thing – what Nigel Slater described as being like wrapped in a cashmere blanket; 'A food so comforting and soul-warming you imagine there is no problem on the earth it could not solve.' Of course, sea-salt porridge seemed the right thing to be eating now I was in Scotland anyway, but I also ordered salmon smoked over whisky-infused chips (took me a while to realise that these related to the smoking process, and not some French fries to accompany my fish) and a potato scone. I was Caledonian in every mouthful.

I also got some *sencha* tea with mallow and sunflower petals and rosebud. It was that sort of place, and with such a breakfast inside me I felt more equal to the city's elegant streets.

I wandered past the (many) cafes declaring that 'JK Rowling wrote Harry Potter here' – as well as the café announcing that 'Harry Potter was not written here' and the place that said that 'JK Rowling possibly wrote Harry Potter here too (probably)'. I found Henderson's, a family-run shop 'passionate about sustainable, ethical food choices' where I bought a shampoo bar and some oat cream for my vegan cooking days.

But mainly among the long boulevards of New Town I found wind tunnels I had to battle down to reach the smart store where today I'd get to experience the legendarily sophisticated (expensive) approach to yoga.

Lululemon is a company which offers yoga clothes with strange names (is 'Align Pant' a series of imperatives or legwear?) and high prices ('Sweaty Endeavor Tight pants' at £88, 'Enlighten Tight pants' at £108, 'Savasana Socks' at £42). It's part of the lucrative and growing worldwide 'athleisure' market which represents seventeen per cent of the entire American clothing market.

It's a company who had said 'Our vision is to elevate the world from mediocrity to greatness', which didn't seem to me to have the ring of yogic truth to it. I'd read an interview with their founder, Dennis 'Chip' Wilson, who explained:

> When we first started, we hired nothing but yogis but it didn't
> work because they were too slow. So we started hiring runners
> who like yoga. They're more on the ball, more type A.

In his book, *Little Black Stretchy Pants*, he writes of how 'each day I walked into the office and asked myself "If I had to compete against Lululemon, what would I do?"'. It sounded paranoid.

'I was fanatical about building a moat around our success,' he admits.

The free classes offered every week at each Lululemon store are part of their USP and presumably a carefully calculated loss leader. I was steeling myself for the 'loss' in a 'Type A' yoga travesty, but as the minutes passed I became aware of just what a 'leader' this was. When I arrived at 9.30, before the shop had opened, I was the first in the queue. Next came Agnes, her daughter and husband, who told me that they all do the class every week – 'It's free – in George Street! Nothing's free in George Street!'

By 9.45 there were over thirty people behind us, sipping at their reusable water bottles. Some were in fancy leggings – the ones with the diagonal strips of mesh wrapping round the legs – but others told me they could never afford to shop at Lululemon and didn't have the budget to do yoga at studios either, but that the free classes gave the chance to practise at least once a week in a group.

So not only the price tags but also the hearts of those at Lululemon were of gold?

Maybe this wasn't the cynical monetisation of yoga I had feared. And I had been aware of a certain bagging in my Primark leggings – indeed in exactly the places I had noticed bagging in my own body. As the material thinned I had been thinking it would be appropriate, not to mention kind to those who'd be standing behind me in future yoga classes, to get a new pair. This could be the place to do it.

Once the shop doors opened I investigated my shopping opportunities, swiping through the leggings hanging around the walls. I just wanted something basic but it seemed I was in the wrong section as all of these were painfully expensive, with elaborate descriptions of their sweat-wicking properties and the textiles they were made from. I approached the sales assistant.

'I'm sorry, but um… could you show me your cheapest leggings?'

She waved a hand to where I'd been looking.

'Those are the cheapest there. Seventy pounds.'

No wonder Lululemon could afford to offer a free yoga class now and then, said a snide voice in my head, unstilled by yoga, and intent on taking a self-righteous stance against Commercialisation and Corporates...

> Success is achieved neither by wearing the right clothes nor by talking about it. Practice alone brings success.
>
> Hatha Yoga Pradipika manual

I went downstairs to the yoga class almost – almost – uncaring about whether I was baggy or not.

The yoga class was to be held in the basement. Initially, its windowlessness bothered me, but I remembered the Pradipika's description of the marks of a yoga hut as described by masters practising Hatha – 'a small door, no windows, no rat holes; ... well plastered with cow dung, clean and bug free.'

With the exception of the dung, this looked like it qualified. A gentle teacher called Jack smiled as she watched us filing into the room where mats were set out in tight rows and columns with literally an inch between them. The room reminded me of busy mosques I'd visited where a geometric design on the carpet also discreetly identified how each prayer mat should be placed in order to maximise the space.

Of course many of the moves we'd be doing this morning were the same that formed part of the Muslim prayer ritual too: Mountain pose to Flat Back, back to Mountain, then Child's pose, Hero pose... When I had been invited to pray with a community in a mosque in Kosovo I had used these familiar names to help guide me through the practice. The woman next to me had even congratulated me on my technique at the end. I would be snuggled next to my neighbour in this morning's class just as cosily as I'd been next to her at that Friday prayers – I counted sixty people settling here onto their mats.

These mats had been provided by the store and were made of tough rubber, like supermarket conveyor belts, and they made a farty noise as you slid palms or feet down them. This was particularly agonising as this was definitely not a class for flatulence: it was a squeeze and intimate. It reminded me of having tried to sleep next to a young Japanese guy on the bus the previous night.

Here I had to jerk my face away when the long-legged man in front of me stretched fully into his Warrior III, and when we lay on our backs and were invited to lower our knees to the right side and turn head to the left I had the option of either lightly resting my knees on my neighbour's left arm or not doing the move at all.

But, like all the best yoga classes, you could still lose yourself here. It didn't matter whether you were on a lake in Nottingham or in the middle of a National Trust site, in your front room, or surrounded by sixty people, it could still be just you and your breath.

Meanwhile, Jack was talking. I hadn't wanted to listen to the kind of spiritual guidance I'd imagined hearing at an athleisure shop – I remembered the Adidas store I regularly passed on my runs with its big 'Type A' poster in the window saying 'I am at my best when I challenge myself. I am never done.' It might (perhaps?) be a philosophy to speed me home, but it promised ultimate frustration, not to say exhaustion.

To my surprise, Jack's soft voice was saying now, 'You are absolutely enough in this moment'. From my Downward-facing Dog I looked back at my feet and saw my ankles were still swollen from the night on the bus. But, I told myself, I was enough.

Jack paced between our mats like a panther in a cage, aware of the power in her beautifully-proportioned body. I'd met teachers before who most of all wanted an audience. 'Look at my abs,' they would say and it wasn't clear whether we were supposed to copy, applaud or just silently envy.

But Jack didn't take us through any virtuoso displays. There were no headstands, no Scorpion or Side Crow. I was right to have sensed her power but it wasn't that kind of power she had – as the class unfolded I felt that her virtuoso gifts were of empathy or love; something you could only call 'positive energy'. It radiated across us all, Sunday-morning slow and not quite comfortable in our bodies.

She led us through inhaling as far as we could, then holding the breath before inhaling a little bit more and finally breathing out. I wished I'd had a chance to brush my teeth at the bus station this morning.

We did it again, and I joined in as Edinburgh exhaled… It was a beautiful sound – like surf in a human ocean. Jack had made us feel connected – to our breath and to each other; to something bigger than us and something even more precious than the pricey leggings sold here.

At the end of the session, I went to talk to her.

'Um, that was lovely!' I said. She looked at me, picking up on the catch in my voice.

'Yeah,' I acknowledged, 'I was expecting it to be superficial. I guess I had Lululemon down as all about what you look like…'

'Yes, they are commercial,' she admitted. 'But doing these sessions is a great way to raise awareness about the community yoga my studio does. It's one of the things I love about the yoga community in Edinburgh – it's so non-competitive and supportive.'

I couldn't see any moats being dug here. She also works at a studio called Shanti Collective as well as at Edinburgh Community Yoga and asked me whether I had picked up a leaflet, so I started to read.

Edinburgh Community Yoga is a social enterprise and the leaflet told me more about their work:

> Our vision encompasses the yogic values of respect and compassion and the humanist ideal of unconditional positive regard.

Yup, with all my preconceptions this morning I had a way to go in putting that ideal into practice.

I read on:

> ECY works with people with mental health conditions, those in recovery from substance abuse, military veterans, women recovering from violence and refugees.

They were shortly to run a fundraiser (over a hundred people doing a Sun Salutation together) aiming at generating the money they needed for their outreach programme through the year. It would be supported by... Lululemon.

So the class really wasn't a triumph of capitalism.

Were there *any* bad guys in yoga?

I took my leave of Jack in a flustered mix of apologies and congratulations, and went to pick up my stuff. My panelled tote bag – big enough to carry my laptop, my flask, diary, book – caught on my foot, and a small tear turned into a rip that completely opened up the side. Glasses case, notebook, purse all spilled out. I gathered it all up, but it was clear that the only way I'd be able to hold my possessions together now would be to cradle them as I walked through the streets of Edinburgh; I needed urgent intervention.

I thought of the shop upstairs and decided I would once again look into the possibility of buying some leggings. They would surely come with a bag. Of course they were expensive, but Agnes had said that they really *lasted*.

Once again I stood at eye level with a multicoloured array of crotches. Seventy pounds! I thought of the woman in that mosque in Kosovo and knew that seventy pounds would feed her for months. I couldn't do it.

The sales assistant saw me thinking about it.

'Can I help you?' she asked.

'I was just wondering about buying your cheapest leggings but all I really need is the bag I was hoping they'd come in,' I said apologetically, gesturing to the jumble of possessions I was gripping in my arms.

'Here, take this,' she said, passing me a lovely tough nylon reusable bag with fabric handles, and printed all over with Lululemon motivational quotes. My favourite:

Meditate for ten minutes every day, unless you're busy – then meditate for twenty.

But also:

Breathe deeply
Do it now, do it now, do it now
Ignore the haters, including yourself
Friends are more important than money

I gave in. Round here, amid the £70 leggings festooning the room, they actually were living the yoga brand.

Gratitude diary entry
that Edinburgh bus station has left-luggage lockers to leave my rucksack in

Chapter 6

Wiped – Hot Yoga and Belonging in Brighton

'When you realise you are the ocean,
you no longer fear the waves'

On my walk from the station through town on a sunny weekend I navigated a rainbow of houses. Where the dominant colour scheme in Edinburgh had been that of the paint which Farrow and Ball call 'elephant's breath', this town was decked out like a village fete, tastefully jolly. The only parts of the neighbourhood which were truly garish were the flowers in the front gardens, bursting out in gaudy yellows and blues, along with the false spring of violet-coloured Cadbury wrappers that passers-by had planted.

According to my directions I was near the yoga studio now, but I couldn't see a sign for the unlikely sounding destination of 'Donkey Mews' (did someone mix up the noises animals make?). As I peered hopefully at building numbers, a girl in her twenties came out of a cupcake-coloured house. She was carrying a Hula-Hoop and I reckoned she'd know where the neighbourhood yoga studios were. In fact she said she'd only recently moved in, but she directed me to the local pallet-wood and chicken-wire juice bar on the corner. Surrounded by lavender plants in zinc pots, of course they'd know where the studio was. And by this time I had no doubt where I was; I had arrived in Brighton.

On a sunny day like this, the town's name seemed the perfect portmanteau word for a place that is *bright* and *right-on*. On my walk to get to the studio I'd seen that here you don't eat just any ice cream, it's vegan ice cream; you don't drink just any coffee, it's 'small batch' coffee. To make your way down the shopping street you don't walk – you skate and glide and roll. The only drunk I had seen was inaccurately trying to put empty wine bottles into a recycling bin.

Combine these indicators with the fact that Brighton had the lowest concentration of 'religious devotion' in England (at fifty-eight per cent) in a recent National Statistics Office survey and it's no surprise that the city was in the vanguard of an innovative yoga form like Hot Yoga. It was at this studio that the first Hot Yoga training was run in the UK and if you want to sample the Hot Yoga approach this seemed like the right place to start.

I opened the door of the studio to a belch of aromatherapy oils. Jan at reception told me gently that I was too late for the current class but that it wouldn't be long before the next one. As I breathed in sandalwood and orange, I felt that simply by having come here I was caring for my body. The feeling increased as Jan gave me directions to the best place for me to wait until the next class – a café nearby with what she said was the best cake in town – and with her response I lurched my heavy rucksack onto one shoulder to leave. She shuddered a little.

'Please,' she said with a smile as if she was in fact offering me a treat rather than making a request, 'could you put it across both shoulders?' It turned out she was a trained yoga teacher herself, used to parsing the world in terms of strain and release, tangled energy lines and misaligned muscle. I felt like she had just given me a hug.

I wasn't able to get a glimpse of the studio where the class was going on so at this point Hot Yoga was still a mystery to me, but even from the reception area I was beginning to understand some of its preoccupations. Along with her recommendations for cake, Jan wanted me to go and drink lots of water. She advised me to bring more water to the class, and her reception area was pinned with signs encouraging yogis to bring their own reusable water bottles for the studio's filtered drinking water, as part of their commitment to being a carbon-neutral business. There were more signs urging us alternatively to buy the bottles of Life Water, which 'deliver 1,000 litres of clean drinking water to a community in need with every purchase'. Another notice was on how to manage cash flow by buying credit at the studio as a solution for those Hot Yoga nightmares – 'Have you found yourself without cash to hand to pay for your isotonic coconut water?'

Perhaps it was the relentless sound of the sea outside, but this water obsession at the studio made me suddenly aware of myself as a being two thirds liquid – a small ocean of gentle tides as fluids sloshed and gurgled into me and drained out. I wished I hadn't eaten a Krispy Kreme doughnut at the station on the way here. Obediently, I went away (rucksack across *both* shoulders) and ate cake and drank lots and lots of water and got back in good time for the class.

Walking into the class later, the heat gave me an instant slap in the face. But it was not sauna-hot – this was humid rather than dry heat. And it was only going to get more humid, I realised, as the nine of us present for the class contributed our evaporated body fluids to the soup. Hot Yoga classrooms are usually between thirty-five and forty-two degrees; I moved slowly and settled onto my mat.

Almost as soon as the class started, my liquid self made its presence felt. I wasn't used to sweating during my yoga practice, and I liked the dry competence of the sequences I usually did. For me, sweating while practising yoga meant you were struggling. Despite this ultra-heated practice room, at the first prickle down my back I felt embarrassed.

I comforted myself that it was not perspiration being *pushed* out of my body by exertion so much as something being *pulled* out by the oven of the classroom. But nevertheless, when the prickling turned to a bead making its way down my spine I was mortified. I knew that sweating was natural; I didn't think I was so oppressed as to believe that women should only 'glow', and yet I felt like I had done something disgusting here, like breaking wind in public.

No matter that I was not the only one starting to gleam – glancing up I saw that the other participants in the class also had slippery skin and damp clothes. As the practice continued, damp became drips; drizzled became drenched. The ocean pounded on outside, and the windows trickled water on the inside. I hadn't realised the experience would be quite so dramatically cathartic; after twenty minutes we were swimming-costume wet. I noticed in the mirror that my white T-shirt was regrettably translucent. Sweat ran down my face, and then we went into Downward-facing Dog splits and the sweat ran back up my face… The burst blister on my foot started to sting with it and my whole body seemed liquefied. When Sharon, our teacher, told us to hold each elbow in the opposite hand behind our backs (if you've never tried to do this, have a go right now and you'll understand that it's more challenging than it sounds), my hands flailed behind me and couldn't grip anything, fingers slithering across forearms like slippery muscular fish which resisted my grasp.

I told myself that other cultures organised opportunities for people to sweat together – from Moorish hammams and Roman baths to Finnish saunas – so this was more normal than it felt. Certainly, the other participants seemed unbothered by turning themselves into human fountains, and by the synchronised pitter-patter of our sweat onto each of our mats. Sharon was even brave enough to come around and offer adjustments to the poses; I imagined her having to take the firm stance of a Turkish oil wrestler to do so with any effective hold.

After an hour of the ninety-minute class she opened a window and fanned us with the door but it was too little too late. Nevertheless, by then I had understood not only the dehydrating impact on my body, but the benefits of the heat in this form of yoga. It was only the second time that I'd been able to get my heels down in Downward-facing Dog.

Sharon had taken us through other familiar poses, including some of those I knew to have been controversially 'patented' by the founder of Bikram Yoga, who created the idea of a practice designed for specially heated environments. Bikram Choudhury is a figure who seems to thrive on such controversy, far from the image of unworldly yogic calm. An energetic man in his seventies who held his classes dressed only in Speedos, headset and a Rolex, Choudhury apparently got the idea for Hot Yoga having practised in his well-heated flat one winter and seeing how the conditions increased the suppleness of muscles. He went on to design a particular combination of twenty-six poses into a script which 'Bikram' teachers have to learn by heart. His clients included three presidents – Clinton, Reagan and Nixon – and celebrities such as Michael Jackson and Jennifer Aniston. Bikram-branded studios had to pay a monthly fee for this privilege – and on the proceeds from the over one thousand studios across the world Bikram lived in LA with his forty Rolls-Royces and Bentleys. That was until the legal costs of challenging allegations of sexual harassment and assault caused Bikram Yoga to file for bankruptcy and Bikram himself to flee the US in 2017.

Nevertheless, even while his appeal as an individual may be turning lukewarm, the interest in his yoga style hadn't cooled. Instead, what emerged was Hot Yoga studios, which use the same principle of the heated environment but without Bikram's script – or the monthly payments to him. Of course he contested the idea of such independence, and the founder of this studio in Brighton is one of those whom he has labelled 'impostors' running a 'Mickey Mouse organisation'. Employing a metaphor that perhaps came naturally to someone who spent their professional life producing liquid, he said:

> These illegals are … diluting my yoga. I win every case: I put them out of business.

But this business seemed to be thriving – along with two studios in Brighton offering Bikram Yoga at the time of my visit, and one other Hot Yoga studio. And here we were thankfully free of Bikram's famous heckling of the yogis he's instructing (one article I'd read reported him shouting at a participant, 'Why you have a fat arse, fat stomach, you been eating too much food?'). Sharon was smiling, encouraging, gentle. 'Practise *ahimsa* – non-violence – to your own body.' She warned us about pushing ourselves too far, and over the course of the class congratulated each of us by name at appropriate points in the sequence. I felt an additional warm glow come over me with the praise for my Trikonasana, and the respect for a good teacher.

Some of the poses we tried in this studio were those in Bikram's series of twenty-six, but then – as opponents to his patent pointed out – these are positions which human bodies have held for five thousand years, so his right to exclusivity is dubious. We did my favourite Dancer pose (which he calls 'Standing Bow'), Eagle pose, Locust, Awkward pose on tiptoes, and what he calls matter-of-factly 'Wind-relieving pose' on our backs with a knee hooked up to the stomach while the other leg is extended. Held on one side, it's the same as the way I naturally lie when I'm going to sleep and I mulled that when rotated to a vertical position it is similar to the pose men adopt standing at a bar stool with one leg bent up on a rung. I would be careful to position myself upwind next time I was in the pub.

There was much else that was familiar, and some other novelties – I tried Elephant pose for the first time, bent over with one hand to the floor below my nose. Also new to me was Cactus pose with legs out to the side and bent at the knee, arms out to the side and bent upwards at the elbow. Perhaps these were the kinds of poses which thrive in a hot climate. There were even some mean mini-Shavasana Corpse poses which I was used to taking only at the very end of a class. When Sharon invited us into the first of these I imagined that the class was over, and sank gratefully into the relaxation. A few breaths later I was awakened and we went on with the sequence. Perhaps this was only appropriate for a discipline that believes in reincarnation.

But eventually it really was the final Shavasana and Sharon talked us through relaxation, inviting us to give thanks for the health and strength of our bodies. It was a good reminder – a quiet moment to appreciate your luck at being alive and well, in the middle of the striving and straining.

But even with the 'cool down' the sweat hadn't dried, and we were asked to place the mats in the 'used mats' pile. As I left the class I saw what looked like a five-litre canister of Lysol which I guessed would be used to swab down every surface.

My own surfaces needed swabbing, and down in the changing room I went to shower. A sign reminded us of *saucha* or the yogic discipline of cleanliness, though the studio had also taken seriously enough their commitment to being carbon neutral to ask people to limit their showers (with the studio's eco-friendly shower gel) to three minutes. Stepping naked past the curtain into the shower area I discovered with a lurch that this was a communal shower, and although it was empty when I entered, as I stood fiddling with the controls under the showerhead I went rigid to hear someone coming in behind me. I had never had a communal shower before. Although I am comfortable being naked with strangers, I get squeamish at nudity with people I know… and after ninety minutes in the company of these women I felt I knew them better than I wanted to here. With rising panic I remembered Sharon calling out her praise; they even knew my name!

Never had I been so committed to carbon-neutrality, and I managed the shower in much less than three minutes.

Once out and wrapped in a towel I was back to feeling great. Did it feel like I'd worked harder just because I'd sweated? I didn't think so – I felt the class's impact deep in my muscles but also in my skin, and I was cleansed and washed out in a way that showering alone couldn't achieve.

While we dressed I even got talking to Sharon and the others. As we chatted, we were all slowly building ourselves up from Corpse pose and nakedness – the snap of elastics, the awkward wriggle into tights and trousers, the click of watch straps reclaiming us. At the lockers there was a sign that requested yoginis, 'don't bring your life into the studio with you' and a suggestion that we should remove our jewellery before class. Now as we re-accessorised ourselves I wondered whether it meant we were returning to life. I'd willingly removed rings and earrings before the class but when I'd discovered that my bulky backpack couldn't even fit into the locker I had felt I couldn't match up to this anti-materialistic programme. The tussle with the locker had seemed like a metaphor, and now as I completed my carapace, putting on my coat, and shrugging on the rucksack for my journey home I sensed I was leaving yoga far behind.

Except that as I climbed up to the station I could feel that my afternoon had changed me. I was tired, but there was a new elasticity – not stiffness – in my legs, and a release in my hip flexors. But there was something else that my afternoon had given me. From Jan's mothering at reception, and Sharon's care for each of us in the class, to the uncomfortable intimacy of the shower arrangements and the chummy changing-room chat, the yoga studio's message to me and to all of us had been that 'you belong'. With the sea roaring as the town's backing track, the liquid tides in me felt that they were uniting with something bigger here; and I remembered something I had once read – that 'when you realise you are the ocean, you no longer fear the waves'.

Gratitude diary entry
'karma' soap from Lush

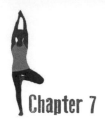

Chapter 7

Doing Time – Yoga in Prison, Surrey

'Right here where you are is okay'

'I suggested we came here because of the doughnuts,' Michael explained when I sat down with him in the Stoke Newington café. 'I came in once and they told me to take as many as I wanted because they were about to close, so now I've made this my regular.'

The world was becoming a kinder place.

My bus had been delayed, and on its way through London two passengers had got into an argument about their rights to reserved seating. Other travellers had joined in. By the time I'd reached Michael I had been late and feeling disappointed with the human race. I apologised to him for my timekeeping, and he smiled a slow gentle smile.

London had not seemed like a home of free doughnuts or smiles as I had been travelling here, and I felt myself beginning to relax.

Which was appropriate because I'd come to talk to Michael about his experience finding and offering kindness and peace in surprising places.

Michael has served three prison sentences for burglary. By the third time he was admitted to jail, he was addicted to heroin.

'Prison saved my life,' he said simply.

He explained how this could be true: how in his cell he found a guide to meditation and yoga.

The booklet was produced by the Prison Phoenix Trust (the 'PPT'), a charity which sends out 2,500 of these books to prisoners every year.

As well as through this literature, their mission of promoting meditation and yoga practice in prison is supported through the teachers they train and the individual correspondence they offer for any prisoner working on meditation and yoga. They're currently helping about 5,000 people in jail, through letters and the 165 yoga classes being run by teachers they've trained in 84 secure establishments.

Their work is part of a growing movement to tackle violent offending with such strategies. A Danish programme, Breathe Smart, uses similar techniques with violent offenders and was recently invited to run a seminar at the Scottish Parliament to share the success of their approach.

Here, among the café's vegan drinks, it all seemed an excellent idea. But then I looked again at Michael and his tattoos and thought about the realities of prison. How on earth had it worked?

'When we had exercise time I'd go onto the grass in the yard and practise,' he explained. 'But yes, it makes you look weird. It makes you vulnerable, and vulnerability is not something you want in jail.'

He had been vulnerable enough as he had also signed up for rehab and was in heroin withdrawal.

Michael wrote to the Prison Phoenix Trust while he was in prison and some of his letters had recently been published by the Trust, along with others, in a book called *Peace Inside*. I asked him about the support he got from these letters and he lit up: 'The people from the PPT are very, very patient. I rejoice in their friendship.' In one letter he wrote 'the feeling of peace, relaxation and release I get from… practice is magical and beats any drug I've ever done'.

Eventually he kicked the other drugs and by then he was regular in 'another habit'. 'Not a bad habit,' he explained. 'Yoga helps me stay in touch with my body.'

I admired him, and particularly because I had been trying to establish a regular meditation practice for the last eight months.

'How do you do it?' I asked, thinking about my daily struggle. He told me about the focus on the breath which is the centre of the Prison Phoenix Trust's approach to meditation. In *Peace Inside*, the Trust's director, Sam Settle, writes of how it sends the message: 'right here where you are is okay'.

> Your breath is the perfect thing to focus on for meditation. It is as natural as the sky and the breeze. It is neutral, as it doesn't tend to stir up strong emotions. It is quiet, and becomes even quieter as you pay attention to it. It is free… It will be with you all your life. And breathing is something we share with many other living things. Best of all, you are an expert at it, because you've been doing it since you first drew breath…
> Breathing quite literally connects inside and outside.

But I'd tried that. And I had spectacularly failed despite having all the resources of my own home around me. The whirl of my mind's thoughts, memories, ideas, problem-solving, curiosity were what Sam Settle likened to 'a carrier bag blown around by the side of the motorway'. I can't imagine how it would be possible in prison.

Michael smiled again. 'There are those challenges in prison too, but one thing is different: you've got time – in prison you've always got time.'

The Prison Phoenix Trust's guide says rather blithely that 'a prison cell can be an ideal environment in which to practise yoga' and Sam pointed out that prisoners' rooms are given the same name as the cells that monks and nuns live in. Somehow Michael – like those 5,000 other prisoners being supported in yoga and meditation – carved out the space to be able to practise. He shrugged, 'I'd just bang on the wall to ask my neighbour to turn the TV down before I started.'

What about the victims of his crimes, I asked. 'Yes,' he said carefully, 'I have to take responsibility for my actions; my practice has helped me understand that. Through a restorative justice programme I met with a woman whose house I'd burgled, and that was a profound experience. Acknowledging what I'd done to her had to be joined up with my loving kindness meditation.'

He'd been out of prison now for over four years and had maintained his 'habit' with meditation every day. And had he joined a yoga group, I ask? He grimaced and said he went to some local ones sometimes but…

'It shouldn't be *Look how bendy I am; look at my yoga pants* or about *having a bit of a stretch*,' he grumbled, 'if it's coming from your ego it's not yoga.' His rigour and discipline made me feel ashamed: ashamed that I couldn't be like him in this – or at least not yet. Ashamed that I had come to this conversation aware of all the things I had which he had not had, and unaware of all that he had which I was missing.

Later in the day I was sitting in a Half-lotus glaring at a flame. Around me my home was quiet, and there was the smell of something relaxing floating out from the candle. There was no good reason why I couldn't focus on the in-breath, the out-breath. But I heard scraps of my conversation in the cafe, the argument on the bus, Michael's neighbour's television, cursing further down the corridor, the sound of doors locking.

And then it came, with a roar like the sound of an inhalation when you are really concentrating on it, and the stillness flooding the body's fibres like the moment of perfect calm before the release of the breath: *right here where you are is okay*. Although the moment passed, it was a tantalising glimpse of what Michael had described as 'magical', and it was enough to keep me looking at the candle, to keep me sitting with the breath, just doing time.

The glimpse made me curious not only to work at my own practice, but to see at first hand how it could work in the challenging environment of a prison. Clearly there were two ways to do that, and I chose what I thought would be the easier one.

It turned out still to be elaborate – before I could visit HM Prison Downview I was sent a list of items I couldn't take in with me. So 'drugs' I could understand. 'Firearms' made perfect sense but 'perfume' was more surprising. 'Chewing gum, wax and associated products' was bewildering until a friend suggested how they could be used to help make an escape. I started thinking like someone deprived of liberty. I worked out that the prohibition against yeast – not something I usually carried in my bag, despite my obsession with nutritional yeast flakes to see me through the cheese cravings of my recent attempts at veganism for a few days each week – was because it could be made into beer. But without the opportunity to take a Kindle, a mobile phone, glass, a camera, or aerosols with me I realised that most of my usual shoulder bag's contents would get me in trouble. I therefore travelled to HM Prison Downview with only a paperback, an Oyster card, some ID and the key to get me back in my home again. Travelling to Surrey across a London increasingly paranoid (*see it, say it, sorted*) about luggage, I felt deliciously light with no rucksack or any bag at all, and ironically liberated as I set off for prison.

At the gate, I was symbolically asked to hand over my ID, but once I'd exchanged my passport for a plastic token, I was *inside*. I was welcomed by Joanne Sullivan from the PE department. She was petite and blonde in a tracksuit and a ponytail that bounced as she talked.

'Is it your first time in a prison?' her colleague asked me as I passed, rather subdued, through the metallic slamming of repeated doors. It wasn't – I'd done voluntary work in four prisons over the years – but it takes more bravado than I had not to be cowed as I was taken through the series of security gates. Nevertheless the comparison with the other prisons enabled me to notice some of the things that were unusual about Downview's atmosphere. I breathed mindfully as we passed through one of the gardens worked by the prisoners, and caught the unmistakable fragrance of lavender. I realised that even though I was coming to take part in a yoga class here, *wellness* was not something I was expecting to find this side of the chain-link fence.

We reached the PE block where I was introduced to Chris Holt, a yoga teacher trained by the PPT and running four hours of yoga a week for the women in this prison. Joanne explained how they'd come to work together after Joanne had contacted the PPT because she was sure of the benefits of yoga; she said in particular that she saw it as an asset to be able to get women into physical movement who might otherwise not come to the gym. 'If necessary we get referrals from the health department for them to attend Chris's yoga.' She estimated that there were about thirty women in the prison who were taking up the offer of yoga classes at some point, though not all were regular.

Together we went into a space that looked like a conference room. Chris laid out mats and we waited for what Joanne referred to as 'the girls' to arrive.

We waited quite a time. 'Apparently roll-call was late today,' Joanne explained to us as her walkie-talkie crackled, and I remembered what Michael had said about how in prison you always had time. I did not feel like I had time – I had a meeting to get to in Reading after this and a train booked after that back to Cornwall. I tried to stop myself checking my watch.

Eventually the women arrived, chatty and smiling. One had a ponytail that jumped like Joanne's. Chris introduced me and my reason for being there and I waited for aggro or suspicion. After all, not everyone relishes the prospect of their Downward-facing Dog being described to the wider public and these women might have good reason to feel that they didn't want notes about this part of their lives taken and shared.

There was a collective shrug and the women focused on taking off socks and stretching out twinges, and the other rituals of fidget and stilling I was used to at the beginning of any yoga class.

Perhaps these women were so used to being observed, assessed and written about that I was only the latest in a long line. Joanne had already explained that the prison housed women serving a range of sentences – for murder to much lighter offences. She had shown me the block accommodating the women who were allowed out on a regular basis – for up to four nights in a row, to spend time with their family, or during the day to do work or volunteering in the nearby town. 'She's just off to her shift in a fast-food café,' she'd pointed out a woman at reception. But some of these yoginis might have been in the system for a very long time.

Or perhaps they were just as unbothered as the yoga practitioners in every other class I'd been in. As Chris led us through the class, we joined in a 5,000-year-old song or dance that was going on around the world. The view out of the window here was worse but the stretch in my hip flexor as I reached upward in Warrior I was the same as it had been in Nottingham, Yorkshire, Edinburgh and Brighton. And it was the same for me as it was for the sturdy woman with the crew cut next to me, and the girl with all the eye make-up next to her.

This session was a reminder of our commonality. The members of the group, including Joanne, were clearly regular practitioners – this was no fad: together we breathed in and out through Sun Salutations and sequences laid down in our shared muscle-memory.

We tried Tree pose and the room shimmered with the instability of our attempts to keep our bent legs high on our supporting thighs. 'When you wobble,' said Chris, 'it's just a conversation between your brain and your body.' I let that dialogue continue. For a while my body won, but eventually my brain got too full of itself and my raised leg trembled back to the floor.

Yoga requires focus and discipline. I didn't know what these women had Done that had led to them being here – just as they, thank goodness, didn't know many of the things I'd done and the mistakes and misjudgements I'd made. But whatever anger, addictions, weakness, pain, poor calculations, fear, loss, betrayals or revenge had led us all to, we moved together in the physical and mental stretches and stamina of Crescent Moon, of Chair pose. As we folded into Child pose, I felt sure that this was part of a journey out of those 'things that no longer serve us' and it didn't seem naïve to feel we would all behave better when we'd learned what yoga had to teach us.

'I don't know whether it's digging that compost heap or yesterday's yoga, but my butt really hurts,' one of the women grumbled as we moved into a stretch. Honestly, and with no disrespect to Cornish villages, we could have been in Port Isaac.

We moved into Cobbler pose, sitting with the soles of our feet together. I had always assumed that the pose got its name from the position you might sit in on the floor if you were working on a pair of shoes placed in front of you. Today I realised that it might be our own feet that we were working at mending.

'Sorry I'm late,' a young woman came in. 'I was working.' Joanne had explained that here everyone had a job, whether helping with the functioning of the prison or at one of the enterprises such as the jeweller and clothes-making business that had been set up to offer training and eventually employment outside once the women had finished their sentences.

We went down onto our mats now for some twists.

'This is more comfortable than the prison beds,' commented one yogini.

Joanne had already told me that she'd seen the benefits of yoga among the prisoners in helping them to sleep. But the comment was significant for another reason too – I realised it was the only time in the whole class that any of us had acknowledged where we were. I wondered whether the women had even acknowledged it in their own heads during the session. Was prison like a constant ringing (a clanging?) in your ears or was it something that you could – perhaps with the help of yoga – learn to drown out so you could hear yourself think, so you could believe that 'right here where you are is okay'?

At the end, and in a rush for my train, Joanne escorted me back to the gate where the official would hand back my passport, as if I'd travelled to another country.

'So how did it compare?' she asked. 'How was it different from the other classes you've attended?'

I took a moment.

'It wasn't different at all! And that is what makes yoga so special.'

Gratitude diary entry
waking to a voile curtain fluttering in a breeze

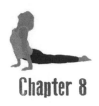

Chapter 8

Smart Cafés with Mismatched Chairs –
Yoga with Asylum Seekers in London

'To increase your success rate, double your failure rate'
Thomas J Watson

At a café run by two women who squabbled in Turkish in the open kitchen, I sipped at a beetroot, apple and ginger juice while I waited for the venue to open for my yoga session. I was in Hackney, in the part of the borough where cafés offer gluten-free brownies and you're seated on an ugly sofa to eat off a requisitioned bedside table with nineteenth-century linenfold carving, and surrounded by a clutter of chairs that don't match.

On the way here I'd passed The Raw Store and a spoon-carving workshop. There were leaflets in Courier typeface offering a 'tasting menu of Hackney-sourced products', and advertising Hackney Herbal, 'a social enterprise that promotes well-being by connecting people with herbs'. There was a 'sling library' and classes for weaving baby yak wool on a SAORI loom. This part of town was like the Middle Ages with the benefit of Wi-Fi.

It was also like a slow-motion – decades slow – international hub. I thought of the maps that airline companies use to show their flights shooting in elegant curved arrows from across the world to their home base, demonstrating the countries they served. If you asked everyone walking down this street to draw their own elegant arrow on a map then you could watch Hackney emerge as a hub over months, years, and generations. When I'd worked at a school here, reading the register had been like reading an index to the world's conflicts and crises. Waves of migration from Syria, from Somalia, from Afghanistan, from the Balkans, from Cyprus, from the Caribbean tracked arrows to this street. Indeed, the most common business on the road where I sat this morning was not cafés offering gluten-free brownies but travel and fashion-bag wholesalers; it seemed to be a neighbourhood always on the verge of moving on or moving out. A neighbourhood of temporary accommodation.

My own arrow to reach here today had been the sleeper train from Cornwall, so it was still early. Through the window of the café I watched Hackney getting itself to work and school. Young women stalked the streets here like dragons, trailing clouds of vape smoke. They held their reusable coffee cups out in front of them like flags, or they cradled the warmth close to their chests like babies.

They all wore shoes with soles that were too high or skirts that were too wide or trousers that were too short or lips that were too orange or headphones that were too large. As a child I had a book that featured Jonas Hanway, said to be the first male Londoner to carry an umbrella. The book had showed him walking through an eighteenth-century London street past houses not dissimilar from those I could see here. In an engraved image a dog lunged at this ridiculous person so egregiously dry in the rain. A family stared and the text had told me that children laughed at him and threw stones.

Looking at these young women's proud newfanglings I felt that Hackney was the spiritual home of all Jonas Hanways. I knew that ten per cent of these outlandish styles would become mainstream next season – and that the other ninety per cent were always going to look just wrong.

But Hackney is a place for seeking out the ten per cent. It's a *start-up, pop-up, incubator, innovation lab*, and *social enterprise*. It's a place of diversity – diversity that inspires you and diversity that threatens to overwhelm you. Diversity brings cultures together in a clash that sometimes looks like a fusion restaurant and sometimes looks like a knife fight. Ten per cent of everything that happens here is salted caramel or other Jonas Hanway 'umbrellas' that soon become part of everyone's landscape because they work.

But, as Thomas J Watson says, the fastest way to success is to 'double your failure rate'. Hackney is a place of people hurtling on what we think is the way to success, and inevitably the failures pile up fast. This is also a place of sink estates, bankruptcies, forced deportations, drugs, slipping through the net – the dreams that didn't work out. On the way here I'd passed a bubble-tea café. For every turmeric latte, successfully combining disparate ingredients in new ways and commanding the prices that could be demanded of the trendsetters, there's a shabby bubble-tea café not quite catching on, not quite paying the rent.

I was visiting a yoga project that was definitely on the turmeric latte side of the line. OURMALA is a yoga project started by Emily Brett, offering yoga to people who are refugees or seeking asylum. Now across twelve locations in the UK, it had started here, at the Hackney City Farm, in 2011. I knew from their website about the evidence they'd collected on the ways that their programme enables refugees and asylum seekers to integrate better into British society and improve mental and physical health. Today was my chance to see their work in practice by joining a class.

By the time I'd finished my juice the farm had opened and I went in to explore. There was a sound of honking from geese across the yard and I hurried on, past the 'Get Loose' bulk store for packaging-free shopping and into the café which was shabby chic in Farrow and Ball and fairy lights; I noticed the first macramé plant-pot holder I'd seen since the 1980s. I was met by Emily.

'You are… just… welcome!' she said, 'I want to give you a big hug.' She smiled, getting up from a meeting with her yoga teacher and an Albanian woman who had just started work with OURMALA as a project co-ordinator.

The project co-ordinator's induction continued. 'When people come for the first time, very occasionally they can be aggressive,' Emily explained the realities of offering something that touches people like yoga does, to people who've had a long hard route to the classes. 'Frankly, it's understandable,' she went on. 'They have suffered immensely, have been let down multiple times and why should they think they can trust us? I have never met anyone in whom aggression has lasted more than a session, though. People pretty quickly understand there's no hidden agenda and the yoga is there to support them, should they find it helpful.' She explained more about the way that OURMALA works, taking referrals from over forty agencies, humanitarian organisations and charities.

Last year across their sites they supported over seven hundred people with yoga. She went through the practicalities: although classes are adapted to ensure that instructions are as simple as possible and assistants are available to help individuals getting used to the class, people coming to OURMALA sessions have to have sufficient English to be able to access the classes, or to have someone who is available to translate should the need arise.

Emily told her story of founding OURMALA, following time on a retreat in India where she accepted a very clear mission of 'devotion in practice'. Returning to London, she started volunteering for the British Red Cross at what was then called the Dalston Destitution Centre. She described the women she met there; all those in her project had been either pregnant or the mothers of very young children and were malnourished from a diet of basic food parcels and the free coffee and biscuits which were often the only other food they could access, handed out to participants at overcrowded English classes.

She started teaching them yoga and saw the difference it made to the women. 'I feel like a human being again,' one of them had told her. When Emily came to Hackney City Farm she was able to expand the initiative, collaborating with the farm to offer to destitute women, survivors of trafficking or modern-day slavery, both access to yoga and also a nutritious meal. Hearing their stories, my night train to get to today's class didn't seem so epic any more.

I'd been told that the yoga class would take place in the Straw Bale Room. I had imagined a yoga studio with some artisanal straw bales posed in a corner (who knew why? It was probably a Jonas Hanway thing. Perhaps we would sit on them instead of *zafu* cushions for meditation?) but when I was sitting on my mat and surveying the room I realised that the straw bales were not in the room. Instead the room was in the straw bales: this was a cob and straw bale construction. In a few places the whitewashing had been interrupted so you could see how it had been put together. I wondered what impression all this made on the refugees who came here. You run from poverty and persecution in Somalia and find yourself in a specially made mud hut in the middle of London.

But it was quite a special mud hut, strewn with Lululemon mats (RRP £38) which were a contribution on top of a £22,000 cash donation from the good guys of commercial yoga to OURMALA's work. And as the class participants settled on their posh mats no-one but me seemed to be wondering at the surroundings. In fact Emily had said that since many new arrivals to Hackney came from rural backgrounds, a visit to a place like this where things grow and geese honk could be a nostalgic experience.

Carolyn was our teacher today. Before the class she'd told me about her training in Scaravelli approaches to yoga (Vanda Scaravelli's defining quote may be that 'Elongation and extension can only occur when the pulling and the pushing comes to an end'). She talked about her interest in yoga as a path to holistic wellbeing, as well as the ways she adapts her usual teaching when she's working with vulnerable people like refugees. 'I don't ask people to close their eyes or leave them alone with their breath,' she said.

Because the needs of the people practising yoga here today would be quite specific, given the trauma many carry with them, OURMALA's teachers are generally asked to volunteer for six months while they and the organisation have the chance to assess whether the partnership is a good fit. After that, their work is paid – though Emily said that some teachers ask for their salaries to be returned to the charity.

Now Carolyn brought us together and led us in some co-ordinated breathing and focus exercises. We looked out past her over the farm's wilderness of hardy allotment plants and chicken wire. Above a fence, buses could be seen passing by and I remembered what my friend had advised me when I started trying to meditate. She'd said that it was not about stopping your thoughts from coming, but that when they came you could marshal them across your mind like clouds across a bright blue sky. I knew that from now on when I meditated it would be scudding double-deckers that I would marshal across a view of rhubarb leaves instead.

Making it even harder to concentrate was the inquisitive squirrel who could also be glimpsed through the window. When I'd read Philip Pullman's fantasy trilogy, *His Dark Materials*, where everyone has an animal daemon who follows them, I'd known that my daemon would be a squirrel. And now here was my attention skipping and scurrying around the possibilities of the community garden when I should have been listening to the sound of my exhale...

The distractions continued as we moved through some familiar *asanas* or poses. I felt the stiffness – the stored tension – in my hips starting to disperse, and remembered once finding myself in tears in a yoga class and the strange but widely-recognised phenomenon of how working on this particular stiffness releases such emotions. I imagined what yoga could make possible for the women around me.

A siren wailed from a police car outside; *let the noises be noises*, I repeated to myself as my meditation tutorial had taught me. I tried not to be distracted by the others in the class either. Although there are forty-three people on OURMALA's register for classes here, today it was a small group and I was surprised that they were older than me. One of them wore a headscarf and from her conversation about Christmas traditions I guessed she might be an Orthodox Christian from Eritrea. I never found out her name but she had been chatty before the session had started, telling me how she loves the yoga classes. 'I not do yoga three weeks; I paining,' she'd said, gesturing at a body made stiff by age, by lack of practice and by who knew what else on its long journey here.

The woman next to me was particularly inflexible. Carolyn invited us to get down on all fours and my neighbour struggled. From my place a few feet away from her, concentrating on my flat back and the line of energy from the crown of my head, I sensed and heard her confusion and flailing. It wasn't just that she found it difficult to follow the verbal instructions we were given; even with the one-to-one support from the class assistant it seemed more that she couldn't remember how to work her body. It was like watching someone battling to erect a deckchair.

Later we were taken into Bridge pose, from which Carolyn suggested putting two foam blocks under our hips. I was usually disdainful of blocks and aids in yoga but, especially after my night on the train, this was delicious; the class sank in unison into a strange cradling. This was a yoga session going just where it was needed.

After the class I walked back to central London; through the evidence of Hackney's new money, from wealthy creatives and city workers, and the evidence of its wealth disparity. 'There's an extraordinary energy here,' Emily had said of the borough and the motivation to start her yoga project here, and my walk took me through streets that can exhaust you with their new ideas, past more smart cafés with mismatched chairs, and through communities made richer and poorer by their endless new arrivals, all bringing their different ways of making the world work. I raised a silent beetroot juice toast – a silent namaste – to all the Emilys, and to all the Eritrean women and others making this a place of opportunity.

Gratitude diary entry
the velvet cushion inherited from my grandfather
that enabled me to get pillowed sleep in my seat on the
night train

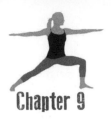

Chapter 9

Yoga for People Living with Parkinson's – West Kilbride

'There's more to this than medication'

'This is what lies ahead; just accept it.'

It could be an expression of yoga philosophy, but Angela McHardy told me that paradoxically it was this attitude, as articulated by the medical profession in relation to her diagnosis of Parkinson's, that was what she set out to fight using yoga.

The limitations that came with her diagnosis were not something she was willing to 'just accept'. As she told me what she did next, her voice quavered with Skype's distortion of the vowels. The computer was doing it to my words too, like contracting a degenerative disease.

'What I was being offered was such a deficit model,' she says, and I heard the experience of a former head of education speaking. 'I wanted something that was beyond the meds approach.'

She could be forgiven for turning to meds, and a duvet and a big bowl of her chosen comfort food because the year she was diagnosed with Parkinson's was also the year she lost her father (who had the same disease) and the year her husband left her.

But instead, Angela turned to yoga. Now a qualified instructor, she spends ninety minutes a day practising and says, 'When I get on my yoga mat, I feel like the Parkinson's really just melts away.' What frustrates her is not having scientific evidence of the impact of yoga for managing the disease.

'But I just know it works,' Angela laments, with the wail of every woman who's ever been told by someone in a lab coat that she doesn't know what's going on in her body – and the desperation of anyone whose body is telling them that time is running out.

'I went to India,' she said, 'and when I came back I talked to my neurological consultant. He's from India, and even he said it: there's more to this than medication.' Since then he has even referred someone who now comes for weekly yoga individual sessions with her.

Because Angela is on a mission. Where other yoga teachers I've spoken to have peppered their talk with Sanskrit, Angela's was more likely to be seasoned with *start-up grants*, the *information hub* she's creating, and something I think is going to be a *one-stop shop*. She's contributed the pay-out she got for her ill health so that soon she'll be hosting classes at her own venue, designed by an architect she knows from when he was a local pupil. She's naming it in honour of her late father's birthplace, Stonehaven, using the Sanskrit word for 'stone'. And when Upala-haven isn't hosting classes it will be a drop-in centre for people living with Parkinson's to learn about available resources, and she's crowdsourcing the funding to hold a series of workshops there about managing Parkinson's. She'll also support the work of Parkinson's Disease Fighters United with money raised from art exhibitions held at the centre.

She invited me to attend one of her classes in West Kilbride. I knew nothing about West Kilbride except for remembering its accolade as once (in 2004) having the highest number of recorded UFO sightings in the UK. The distinction has since passed to Bonnybridge, fifty miles away on the other side of Glasgow, now the 'World UFO Capital'. But I discovered that more recently the town has moved on from an association with spacecraft and reinvented itself with a focus on a different kind of craft. Angela's classes are held in the award-winning Barony Centre which I read is part of West Kilbride's self-styling as Craft Town, for which it won the Enterprising Britain competition in 2006. I could see Angela and her attitude fitting in fine.

Arriving at the Barony I was met by a crowd of local faces. Just the faces though – the frozen stares of masks, made in one of the town's craft projects, which were mounted on the walls. Once I'd realised what exactly was looming out of the gloom at me I was able to read how the community art project had created replicas of local volunteers in plaster of Paris. Unsmilingly, they continued to watch me as I walked to the room where our class was due to begin.

They reminded me of one of the signs of the devastation Parkinson's can wreak – the so-called 'Parkinson's Mask' which can result as the lack of motor control extends to the facial muscles. I knew a bit about Parkinson's from watching deterioration in several dear family members as well as friends. Fifteen per cent of those with Parkinson's have a family history of it so the sympathy for my relatives wasn't entirely altruistic. This tremulous monster might be lurking somewhere in the body I was taking such care to keep well – like a rather shy but extremely persistent burglar under the bed, ready when I was looking the other way to strip me slowly of my handwriting, my balance, my smile…

Thinking like this was presumably exactly the 'deficit model' that Angela had said she was resisting. I stiffened my spine and opened the door to the class. It was a small group – half a dozen of us settling onto our mats. Not everyone was living with Parkinson's, but I had the chance later to talk to some of those from the class who were. Janice, fifty-two years old and diagnosed with Parkinson's eleven years ago, said of these Sunday night yoga sessions simply: 'It's what's kept me going; it's what's kept me upright.'

Not that any of us found it easy to stay upright. The yoga class seemed to make no concessions to Parkinson's, and I felt the familiar tug at muscles as we worked through Sun Salutations. When Angela invited us to hold ourselves horizontal in Plank I felt a judder and a shudder working through my body and wondered whether Angela was aware exactly what kind of a leveller she had asked of us all.

We moved into Triangle and I struggled as always with keeping my body in a single plane. There's some complicated maths about the angles at which to hold yourself in this pose and I later discovered it was the perfect West Kilbride yoga asana. This town where I was currently folding myself over my extended front leg was the birthplace of eighteenth-century mathematician Robert Simson for whom the Simson Line is named (yes, you've remembered correctly – the line 'containing the feet P_1, P_2, and P_3 of the perpendiculars from an arbitrary point P on the circumcircle of a triangle').

Angela took us through the physical implications of such mathematics with competence and a smile. There was little sign of what my brilliant Uncle James told me of at a family party as his experience of the disease – *you stumble a little and mumble a little and fumble a little*. I wondered at what neurological trick was being pulled here, that enabled her to keep such focus and physical control in ways that were challenging in the rest of her life. I remembered a friend telling me about someone they knew who had Parkinson's and yet could make ships in bottles, using some unknowable reserve of concentration to keep the tremors at bay for this precise focus only during the time when the little contraptions of balsawood and thread were launched.

We were taken through some twists, like the 'bind' where your right hand slides across your back to tuck round the left-hand side of your waist, which I recognised as exactly the move I had to make to catch hold of the second shoulder strap of my rucksack when I was sliding it into place on my back.

Each of her classes has a theme, which Angela calls a 'challenge for the mind' as well as for the body. Tonight it was 'Slow it down'. I thought of the eponymous song by my favourite Scottish singer-songwriter, Amy Macdonald:

> I guess I've been running round town leaving my tracks,
> burning out rubber,
> Driving too fast but I've gotta slow right down.

Like holding Plank, this was a good challenge whether you were living with Parkinson's or not. As we breathed in (sloooowly) I saw why Janice spoke of Angela being not just literally *inspirational*. I could also see the power of having a teacher fighting the same battle that you are.

'You don't feel awkward if you're having a bad day,' Janice said.

Angela heard her and joked back, 'And when the teacher falls over it's alright.' Another woman with great reflexes snapped back, 'We'll try and catch you.'

It was a powerful exchange. It was not just the instinctive offer of support that struck me; it was the plural form she used.

This was the exact opposite of the guru tradition; this was what it looks like when a teacher owns and celebrates her frailty; and this was the empowerment that all the class experienced as a result. I felt that here in West Kilbride I'd gained a significant understanding not just of yoga for people with Parkinson's, but of yoga for anyone.

Gratitude diary entry
the sound of rain

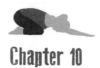

Chapter 10

Upwardly Mobile – Aerial Yoga in Godalming

'Not sure whose green Primark zip-up hoody I borrowed
today for shoulder mounts but I've brought it home to wash.
Will bring it back nice and clean on Tuesday.'

Ironically, I did not have high hopes of my aerial yoga class. For all
that I had had to type in 'GOD' as the station code when buying
my ticket to Godalming, and was setting off on a Sunday morning
for an experience that should raise me up in at least some way, this
felt like a gimmick after the thoughtful approaches to yoga I'd been
learning about. From the map and the website I knew that my session
was to be held in a warehouse on a small industrial estate. As well as
aerial yoga you could learn pole dancing in the same space. I didn't
know much about 'pole' but it carried connotations of meretricious
power without responsibility, movements wriggling out of their true
intention, in the exact opposite of the joining together of movement
and intention that I'd been earnestly practising in my yoga classes.

As I walked through the town to get to the class it was clear that
this was an upwardly-mobile community in many senses of the word.
I had already read that in 1881 it was the first place in the world to
have a public electricity supply and electric street lighting. I passed
small companies based in what would then have been working-class
houses now offering nonessential services, or businesses like dog
walking and garden landscaping as monetised versions of what the
houses' original owners would have considered 'living'. I also passed

the Wilfrid Noyce Community Centre, and a bit of curious googling about its name revealed a more significant way in which a local man had been upwardly mobile – the eponymous Noyce had been on the 1953 ascent of Everest.

The High Street beamed with pride in brand Godalming: little imagination had been used up in naming the shops, as if nothing more were needed as proof of quality than geography – the town boasted The Godalming Shoe Shop (since 1925), The Godalming Butchers, The Godalming Food Company, Godalming Tailors, Godalming Delights (artisan ice cream), and The Godalming Travel Co. The definite articles somehow put the seal on their self-satisfaction.

I went on past the church (where a signboard announced that a lichen found growing on gravestones here was nationally scarce) and continued past Waitrose (where pre-washed salad bags probably included nationally scarce lichen), an oyster bar and an estate agent where a modest 1970s house was being advertised for half a million pounds. It was not surprising to learn that two years ago this town had been rated as the most prosperous in the UK.

The buildings thinned out, and the land got cheaper – though not for long: I passed a construction site promising to be soon transformed into a 'luxury gated development of homes, apartments and coachhouses'. For now, the place was inhabited only by wood pigeons and wild mallow. Round the corner was the entrance to the small industrial estate where I found the Fitness Hangout.

Walking into the studio was like walking backstage at a theatre. There was the same daunting mixture of fairy tale and fire hazard – a place swagged in silk, in the middle of which, like a health and safety inspector briefly allowed into the seraglio, a practical body stood on a ladder checking carabiners.

Each swathe of material hung above a mat, and women were taking their places each at one of the mats. I wondered which of the half-a-million-pound homes they had come from, but they were reassuring to look at; they looked a bit like me – of similar age and build – but just better. They didn't have the Instagram yoga bunny look that I knew was unattainable for me unless I had a skeleton transplant – they were strong and supple and I could imagine that one day, with a lot of effort, I could be like them. I particularly liked Ruth, who had a bag saying 'I do yoga because punching people is frowned on'. Immediately I spotted the one with blue hair and tattoos. There had been at least one woman with blue hair and tattoos in every yoga class I had attended. This felt like increasingly familiar territory.

There were nine women in the room and they all used each other's names as they chatted. One was getting married and they swapped suggestions for wedding-day make-up. I was reluctant to join in. Then someone started a conversation about failing eyesight and I itched to mention the 'fist monocle' trick I'd been using where you can make small print more visible just by viewing it through your curled fist. Maybe I could be a part of this group?

And conversation moved on; the women exchanged stories of having used a yogic 'neti' pot for flushing out the sinuses with salt water and, less alarmingly, about the pub the previous night. Someone was sharing a recipe while another was telling the group how she was supposed to be moving to London but she didn't want to because she'd miss this class. As I listened to this hive mind in action I started to understand why.

Up above us were aerial hoops as well as the poles for the other classes offered at the Fitness Hangout; in the changing area I'd seen a small Buddha statue next to a plaster of Paris high-heeled Pleaser shoe such as I assumed might be worn by a pole dancer. I'd been around enough Buddhas recently to find this an uncomfortable juxtaposition.

But I took my place in the steel forest of poles, positioning my mat by copying what I saw others doing. The woman next to me saw me checking:

'Is it your first time?' she asked. When I admitted that it was – adding defensively, *for yoga, no, but for aerial yoga yes* – she pulled a face. Thinking about it afterwards I realised it was quite a lot like the involuntarily expression pulled when your face is upside down.

'You're going to feel it in your core,' she said, half as a warning and half as a brag.

She was right. Once the class started it seemed that every move we did, or pose we held, involved a tussle with gravity. We were on the mat raising various parts of our bodies up to the cradle of the hammock; we were in a backbend off the hammock and then pulling up to seated, we were seated and clambering up to standing.

Like the floaty silks and the carabiners, it was the combination of the sense of weightlessness and finding some steel in your core or upper body that made the class addictive. It gave you a feeling of grace at the same time as power – perhaps like wearing a sari and knuckledusters. The hammock itself was deceptive – the whispering fabric became as tough as an acrylic rope round your wrists or the top of your thighs, the way a light plastic bag can bite into your hands when loaded with shopping. We might start lazily swinging on our hammocks like the little boy in the Dreamworks ident, but before long we were clambering around like toughened sailors on a man o' war. Or if we discovered that we didn't have those muscles and that strength, we were instead wistfully sitting out that part of the session.

While I sat watching, like the pupil with a sick note, one woman went upside down. Her T-shirt flipped up as she did so, revealing what I would have expected to call her tummy. But it was nothing like a tummy; these were Abs: rippling and taut and wholly unattainable. I was just pleased that I'd thought to wear a fitted top so no-one would see what was underneath it, even if I ever turned upside down.

I spent most of the class desperately disorientated, dizzy and confused. *Up* became *down* as you suspended yourself so even ordinary instructions ('put your arms over your head') made your head spin. And then you spun, too, so that left and right all merged into one. And for some of the class we'd been asked to create small cocoons or what the teacher called 'pouches' out of our hammocks so that I couldn't even see either the teacher or any of my fellow students to copy their movements. Suspended like knobbly quinces swaying from a metal tree, each pulling the orange silk around us to screen out the world, the teacher's use of 'front of the class' or 'back of the room' stopped making any sense as my little pod gyrated. Parting the silk to look out unbalanced me so that I swayed even more.

The blur, as the room spun with my unwinding silk hammock, and the glow – whether of blood vessels seen with closed eyes or of the studio light coming to me filtered through the orange silk – colour my memory of the class. There were precise moments I can remember: wrapping the hammock like a nappy between and behind my legs held in the diamond of Cobbler pose followed by the pounding and then popping in my ears as I allowed myself to lie back and hang down like one of a funky colony of orange bats. Or when we all stood on our hammocks, pulling the silk at the sides in opposite directions like the harmless bows of little Cupids.

We became bows ourselves, too, in a modification of the classic yoga pose, done on your stomach on the ground – the boring old static, supportive ground. Here we did a back bend, supported by the hammock, and then stretched out our arms to find our ankles. Or we tried. There was One-winged Dove and Diving Eagle pose. We used the hammock to support us in Plank, legs on the hammock and core muscles stabilising not only my quavering upper body but also the oscillations of the hammock.

Back in our cocoons we stretched, first in a Child pose, suspended in these temporary wombs, just like the bundles that the stork brought. Then the teacher directed us to bend our knees in a position I was trying to get both my head and my knees around, while making my carabiner creak. From one side came a prompt from the neighbour who'd scared me with her warning about my abs, muffled through the layers of our silks. 'It's like Pigeon,' she said, and I saw at last what the teacher had been trying to get me to do, and managed to move myself into something approximately like the position. I tried a grunt of thanks, but I wasn't sure my neighbour could hear me.

I was ready for the class to end, feeling motion sickness and wearied in muscle and mind. But I also wanted to come back; I wanted to get better at this. I'd been branded by the practice; the next morning, every time I went to do ordinary daily moves – the bending down to pick something up, the pulling on of leggings – my core muscles screamed and I swore. I wondered whether this was what the verb 'Godalming' meant; I certainly spent a lot of time Godalming before the pains subsided. I thought about the woman whose T-shirt had slipped during the class and wondered how many years she'd spent Godalming before she'd sculpted a shape and strength like that.

I was kept in the embrace – a silken but strong hold – of the women I'd joined here in other ways too. I was added to their Facebook group, open only to students, automatically after the session and had the chance there to see how this surprising community on the edge of a Surrey industrial estate built additional real, meaningful muscle. Even after I'd long left Godalming behind, my phone would buzz with a notification of another exchange in the 'hive'. One day the online conversation turned to complimenting yourself and I got to read an articulation of some of what I'd glimpsed in the tough knot of women who'd sailed and swooped and swung in the room with me that Sunday.

'I performed pole on my own in front of an audience yesterday for the first time... I was crying to my boyfriend the night before because I didn't want people to see me in my bra and pants and laugh at 'the fat pole dancer'. I can dance. I am flexible. I look good and I keep proving myself wrong – I can do anything,' wrote Lorna Nye.

Another day the group chatted about the impact of their aerial experiences. One woman wrote: 'I have bad lower back pain; when I leave class it goes away for a while! Nothing else has been able to help it so far.' Others were not aerial yoginis but from the pole group who had so scared me. Laura Johnson wrote 'pole helped me overcome anxiety and find somewhere to fit in'. Sarah Jo Jo Manton wrote of how the group was 'accepting of all, even autistic girls can fit in'. Samantha said pole had got her 'out of depression and fatigue caused by my medical conditions. You cannot compare poling and the sistership and camaraderie to any other form of exercise that I have done. Really brought me out of that dark place.' Bex Burrow said 'it's been a great way to make friends, which is something I can't do easily. But most importantly for me, it's restored so much of the confidence I used to have before being in a rather unhappy abusive relationship. Those scars are hard to mend, but I've finally found somewhere to help me fix them.' The comments were painful but triumphant and they were greeted with hearts studded across the screen like hugs of support.

These are the people I had dared to call meretricious?

I hadn't had to overcome any of the challenges that these women had identified, but I was becoming convinced that if I had had to, it was places like this that could help me through.

The day I really fell in love with Godalming was a much more prosaic Facebook post, though: 'Not sure whose green Primark zip-up hoody I borrowed today for shoulder mounts but I've brought it home to wash. Will bring it back nice and clean on Tuesday!' Lending something to someone you know only as one of your own, or borrowing something and making it better before you give it back, that's a community held at least shoulder high!

So this was a yoga community I was surprised to find myself wanting to return to. The exhilaration of anchoring yourself upside-down was part of it, but the greatest source of the power I found in Godalming was its people, making a community that was behind you, around you, beneath and above you.

Gratitude diary entry
the red purse a friend made me

Chapter 11

Downward-facing Doga –
Yoga With Your Dog in Shoreditch

'Say Yes'

I was in a high-ceilinged Victorian public building with terrible acoustics. In what should have been a quiet time there were shouts and scampering and other forms of off-task behaviour. I looked around, bewildered, and then I heard the voice of Julia saying authoritatively, 'Come *here!*' Some of the noise died down and one of the scamperers returned to her place.

It could have been a scene from my year as a newly qualified teacher in a tough inner London school. Julia had had the classroom next door, with only a partial wall between us. As noise levels rose on an afternoon when there had been wet playtime or some other pedagogical disaster, I became increasingly aware, with each additional decibel, of her presence on the other side of that partition. With all her experience she was a constant source of inspiration, of envy, and – when necessary – of policing.

But today we were not in a school with misbehaving children but in Shoreditch's Passmore Edwards bequest library, now converted into a performance space. And it was not Year Five children capering around the room but dogs.

Julia and I were at a session of Dogamahny™ dog yoga where a dozen people stood in Warrior II trying to modify their breathing while their dogs humped other yoginis, peed in the middle of the room or otherwise ran amok.

We were here because of Julia's New Year's Resolution, to say 'Yes'. Crikey!

As if she had heard her name being called, a dark silken-curled Cockapoo trotted up to me and started sniffing.

She had indeed known she was being called: this was Julia's exquisitely-named dog, Ms Crikey Barker. I had only met her once before, and not having a natural rapport with dogs I'd therefore been a little nervous about her being my yoga partner today. But Julia wrote to me in a message before the session, 'if she eats one of the other dogs, we'll just have to pay their vet bill is all. But she probably won't.'

It was the same kind of reassurance she had offered when I'd been fretting about those Year Five kids.

In the time (over twenty years) since I was a Year Five teacher, Julia and I had lost touch. Then Julia's quest to say Yes led her by a chance link online to something I'd published, and she wrote to me and we were back in contact. But it was more fun now because our conversations no longer consisted of me saying earnestly 'but the National Curriculum says…' and Julia replying, 'oh, you don't want to worry about that'.

In our early Messenger exchanges we played 'spot the difference' over those twenty years of changes. I'd started writing; she'd started working as an educational psychologist. I'd moved out of London. She'd had children, remarried – and recently lost her husband to cancer. So now – this year – she was 'saying Yes to life' and as we strained into Crescent Moon next to one another and a dog weed on my yoga mat, I wondered whether and exactly how this was helping her.

But all of us here were busy saying Yes to life. Why else would you come on a Saturday morning to stand on one leg in a draughty rehearsal space while a dog did her best to unbalance you? There were about a dozen of us who'd said Yes to this particular aspect of life today – a couple who worked at Battersea Dogs Home and said they 'just love dogs'; a woman with a tireless chocolate lab puppy who had introduced him by saying only 'he's been awake and exercising for two hours now and yet still...' when she was cut off by a dog who clearly didn't like the word 'still'; a guy who loved dogs but had never done yoga before; a mother and daughter who'd received tickets for the session as a birthday present; a woman whose terrier patrolled the class with a relentless bark and whom she never let off the lead, despite the teacher's invitation to 'say yes' to the chaos the owner promised would ensue.

Shoreditch was a great place to say Yes. On the street where the class took place I had walked past a shop and café selling real ostrich-feather dusters and where a group of women sat breastfeeding over herbal tea. Yes! I said, to the beautiful feather dusters (£25 though), to the beautiful women, and to the fragrant brews that sat on the table. I'd passed a ping-pong cocktail bar (Yes!), the National Centre for Circus Arts, a night club with a swimming pool, and a fancy-dress shop offering outfits for hire 'by the week, from superheroes to fruits and vegetables'. Yes, yes, yes.

The teacher for our session today was Mahny. She had a body like a bullet and a love of what I was later to discover was Kundalini-style yoga so that as well as managing our dogs and the alignment of our front foot we were led in panting 'breath of fire' as we held poses for upwards of a minute.

She started us sitting cross-legged on our mats with an alarming round of 'If you're happy and you know it, clap your paws' which the humans gamely sang along to while most of the dogs looked on disdainfully.

Then we were invited to focus our breathing. By now I had learned how to do this in my meditation practice. I had described my first attempts at meditation as being like 'letting a puppy out to play' as my thoughts romped around, dug up bits of my mental garden and wagged energetically at irrelevancies. Now I more often had the thoughts under control. They were not yet – and may never be – highly trained gun dogs, remaining calm even under fire, but they could generally come to heel.

As I attempted to focus today, I watched my simile come to life. Dogs careered around the mats, bounded up to the bowls of water left for them in the middle of the circle we had formed with our yoga mats, splashed it on the floor as they drank, trampled their paws in the spillage and leaped off to another corner of the room. Two started play-fighting; others got into something more intimate. There was yapping and squealing, and the suppressed swearing and apologetic fluttering of the hands of owners, and Mahny assuring us all that we should stay just where we were, and that the dogs would sort it out. In previous meditation practices I had been told to 'observe my thoughts', and watching the melee in front of me now felt like I was doing just that.

Mahny was unbothered, 'there will be barking; there will be widdling, there will be humping,' she murmured gnomically.

'I don't have a plan,' she told us cheerfully, and invited us to go with the flow, following her as she was prompted by what she judged to be the energy levels of the humans and the dogs in her class. Some of the dogs quieted eventually, and we yogis held Boat pose with our dogs (our 'dogis') on our laps; we stood in Triangle pose with our dogs under our arm 'like a handbag'. We folded over into Uttanasana and were invited to bury our faces in our dogs settled below us; Crikey's paws paddled into the tops of my feet. We did, of course, hold Downward-facing Dog, and one obliging spaniel mimicked the pose like a guide. We relaxed into Child's pose and for those who were – together with their dogis – willing, Mahny helped settle dogs on people's backs. We stood in Tree without our dogs, though – as when Julia came down from the pose 'like a lumberjack', as she described it, and we heard a squeaking rebuke to her for catching Crikey's tail – the dogs could get involved at all times. Later, rocking backwards enthusiastically on my mat, I almost collided disastrously with something small and furry.

Towards the end we were invited to swap our dogs, and those who had no pet with them held out beseeching arms for Crikey to jump into. I sensed an unfulfilled yearning around the room from those who had come without a dog, the feeling of being full of love and having nowhere to lavish it. This was actually the second time I had tried to come to Mahny's Doga session and on the first attempt the class had been cancelled, not for lack of interest from dog lovers but for lack of interest from dog *owners*: Mahny had explained that the class then wouldn't work because too many of those who'd booked did not have a dog.

I hadn't noticed until today how inner London is a largely dog-free zone. All the challenges to keeping a dog here (space for walks, tenancy agreements...) meant that there were lonely people across the city who were waiting for some way to let wet noses and wagging tails into their lives. On my way to the class I'd kept an eye out for dogs, trying to learn the city through their eyes, their paws. But I saw none. Finally I spotted a woman walking a terrier whom I shadowed for a block or so, only to realise that they were heading to my Doga class. Apparently without such specific invitations (and one woman attending the class had travelled in from Kent), Shoreditch streets were not a place for dogs. Listening then to the busy thrum of this city I heard in it a throb of something sadder – beneath the laptops were laps waiting for the warm bulk of a sleeping dog; in the expensive boutiques girls who were fingering fabrics really wanted to be scratching at a different kind of satin coat.

Mahny had clearly done some similar dog-love arithmetic, and had established that a certain amount of beloveds (dogs) had to be present to balance out the equation for any given number of unrequited lovers (yoga practitioners). Today we had achieved the necessary equilibrium.

To close the session, we lay on our mats and Crikey curled up next to me. After Shavasana was over (*'namaspaw'*, Mahny saluted us all), Julia and I took the dog and our newly-worked muscles out into the world. As a dog owner, Julia already knew but I felt new pride in what we had with us tugging at the end of the lead.

I was curious (Yes!) to sample one of the few things I knew about Shoreditch – the 'cereal cafés' which were the target of 'anti-gentrification' protests about the area a few years previously. The first we found advertised 'Sugar Puffs or Frosties?' at the door, but inside we found that the only cereal on the menu was in fact porridge.

While I spooned my (coconut milk – obvs) porridge, I watched Crikey at work again. It was a very inactive kind of work, because all she did was lie at our feet, but every passing customer or waitress stopped to touch her, to compliment her, to baby-talk her or rub at her like a lucky charm.

I knew that there had been a rise around the world of dog cafés – places that you can go to take up visiting rights on other people's animal companions – and watching Crikey's impact on Shoreditch's endorphins I realised that the Doga class this morning hadn't been what I'd thought it was. This wasn't just hipsters of Shoreditch wanting to say Yes to a quirky combination – which happened this morning to be yoga and dogs but could just as well have been typewriters and iPhones or banana and turmeric (the surprisingly delicious smoothie I had at the café). People were demonstrating that they wanted to say Yes to nuzzling; *yes* to the energy of a puppy; *yes* to enthusiastic welcomes; *yes* to following up interesting smells; *yes* to touch when you're feeling lonely; *yes* to the sound of another creature's breathing next to yours; *yes* to trust; *yes* to play.

Yes.

Gratitude diary entry
the exfoliating mitt I was given for Christmas which makes
me feel shiny, clean and new

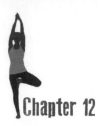

Chapter 12

PraiseMoves – a 'Christian Alternative to Yoga' in Peterborough

'We want to provide a place where you can encounter God,
as well as build friendships with others'
Peterborough Cathedral website

In 2016, a school in the state of Georgia that had been offering yoga to children was forced to withdraw some elements of the programme, such as saying 'namaste' or putting their hands to their heart centre, following concerns about 'religious' teaching. The Alabama Board of Education has banned yoga completely. In 2017 *The Sun* reported that the community centre which forms part of a church in Wales was going to allow Pilates classes but not yoga because 'activities that might be seen to be in conflict with Christian values and belief would not be appropriate'.

Not only Christians but Muslims have also seen yoga as a challenge: in Indonesia a fatwa was pronounced in 2009 against any Muslim practising yoga.

Debate continues in the blogosphere – I discovered that googling 'Can Christians…' brought up '… do yoga?' as the very first in a list of questionable behaviours about which internet researchers have clearly been looking for guidance (other worries were about eating pork, being cremated, drinking alcohol, swearing, marrying non-Christians and getting divorced).

The concern has not been all in one direction – there has also been a rise in criticism of the cultural appropriation that goes on when a Western culture takes over one part of a practice that began in a completely different context. A A Gill described doing yoga for exercise as being 'like walking the stations of the Cross as aerobics'. Rhik Samadder in *The Guardian* developed the simile – it's as 'if all the Hindus in Uttar Pradesh were shovelling down communion wafers as a low-cal alternative to crisps'.

American Dr Laurette Willis answers the 'can Christians do yoga?' question definitively:

> These are postures that are offered to the 330 million Hindu gods. … If you do these postures and you do this breathing technique and this meditation, then you will be accepted by a god, little 'G.' That's the real danger.

Her suggested substitute is a programme she has devised, called PraiseMoves, 'the Christian alternative to yoga', and I discovered that I could sample a class in Peterborough.

The city is fertile religious ground, supporting not just the new KingsGate 'superchurch' which can seat up to eighteen hundred worshippers, and where the PraiseMoves classes are held, but the cathedral – on a site which has held a Christian church since AD655 and where the present building was begun in 1118 – as well as a number of mosques, a Sikh temple and a Hindu mandir.

The cathedral occupies a site rather more central than KingsGate's out-of-town location near the supermarket and I went there first to try to understand its ways of straddling the faith communities. 'Our church is for everyone, and we hope you feel welcome whatever your age, background, or culture. We want to provide a place where you can encounter God, as well as build friendships with others', I was told on the website when I looked for opening times.

Arriving in Peterborough and walking to this faith centre from the station, I passed a strange memorial to one of Peterborough's most famous and inspiring daughters, Edith Cavell, who attended Laurel Court school within the cathedral precincts. Famous for her rejection of jingoism and her desire to have 'no hatred or bitterness for anyone', even on the eve of her death by firing squad in Belgium during World War I, her openness to others seemed to have been commemorated with faint praise in what is presumably the 'Patriotism is not enough' section of the multistorey car park that bears her name.

From there it was not a surprising journey to the Starbucks (St Arbuck's?) on the site of a chapel dedicated to St Thomas Becket, completed shortly after his murder in 1170 and built for the pilgrims venerating the saint's relics which had been brought here from Canterbury.

It was a relief to get away from such latter-day saints and into the cool and calm of the stone glades created by the cathedral's repeated arches. It's a good place of sanctuary, especially for a female writer, because of the history of the monastery which was here until the Reformation and which contributed significantly to the Anglo-Saxon Chronicle. The Peterborough Chronicle is one of the few surviving first-hand accounts of English life of the time written in English, and when it ended in 1154 no chronicle was written in English for three hundred years. It is this Chronicle which contains the first ever use of the English feminine pronoun 'she'. This is where we were written in, girls!

While I was here I also wanted to see the most famous She of Peterborough Cathedral – buried here at her death in 1536, her tomb was then destroyed during the Civil War, though her body was undisturbed. In 1893 the *Daily Mail* invited readers sharing her name to each subscribe a penny. The Kates and Cathies and Kathryns of the day hurried to do so, and enough money was raised to pay for the marble slab which now marks the grave of Catherine of Aragon. The affection in which she is held is shown by the pomegranates, her symbol, left on the tomb. I read this in the guidebook but couldn't quite believe that I would see it. It didn't seem a very English – a very *Peterborough* – thing to do. Even if one wanted to leave a tribute, in the middle of East Anglia, where on earth would one get a pomegranate to leave? Well, six people had found one, and together with some brittle flowers the little offerings sat loyally on the tomb, like four-centuries-old apologies.

I wandered round the rest of the cathedral, trying to guess what it would have to say about yoga, or about PraiseMoves. As the note on its website had suggested, it was working hard to be welcoming and relevant. A table held leaflets about quitting smoking, advice from Age UK, a leaflet in Hindi about looking after your heart… It seemed that this was not just a shrine to dead queens, or a home for precious manuscripts, but a centre for a community.

Next stop on my ecumenical Peterborough pilgrimage was the Hindu mandir. It was the first time I'd been to a temple in the UK, and the first time in over a decade that I'd been to a temple anywhere. Knowing that I'd be going on to the PraiseMoves class and would be in 'yoga pants' ('PraiseMoves pants'?) with bare arms, I had wondered whether this might cause any dress-code problems and had thought I should ring the temple in advance to ask.

The phone had been answered by a woman who, it emerged, was temporarily acting as the temple priest. She was thankfully unbothered by the idea of being able to see my arms or the shape of my legs. 'But,' she added, 'we do ask women not to attend for five days from the start of their period.'

Sometimes you have no idea of the ways you might cause offence.

And this raised an interesting question. No-one but me (and a God or gods I don't believe in) would ever know whether I had my period. If a tree falls in the forest and nobody hears it, does it make a sound? If an ovum falls in the Fallopian tube and nobody knows it, does it make a sin?

I went along anyway. The taxi from the centre of town took me out past Polish shops, Lithuanian shops, shisha cafes, and then we were out to the streets where buddleia grew in neglected front yards.

I asked the driver about the communities here as I was intrigued to know whether PraiseMoves was capitalising on a general intolerance for other cultures. He seemed to find the question baffling, and said his father had been in Peterborough since 1958 while he himself arrived from Pakistan in 1998. According to him relationships between the communities here were fine.

He got me to the temple before it opened so I went to wait at a nearby café. It looked generic, with a coffee menu and a few boxes of herbal tea bags and some cakes. I saw someone behind the counter chatting on FaceTime and my ear attuned. He was speaking Albanian, which I can speak fluently. 'A je shqiptar?' I asked, and we were off.

I asked him, too, about the relationship between communities here, knowing that Albania is marked for its religious harmony between Muslims and Christians. He said the city is just divided geographically – 'you don't see many English people coming to this business. If this street had a more better reputation we might get more better clientele.' But no, he'd seen no racism.

After I'd finished my tea I went back to the temple. It's on the same street as the Samaritans and the soup kitchen – a little haven for the down-at-heel or the down-at-heart. I was given the same welcome I imagined would be extended to the hungry and the hopeless, by the woman I had spoken to on the phone. She was busy preparing votive lamps and offerings on *thali* trays. As she set out ghee and cotton wool twisted into wicks, she told me about the worshippers who attend, mainly from India, Kenya and Uganda. One man who came in was happy to get talking to me and said he was born in Uganda to parents from India. Like my taxi driver, and having been in Peterborough for thirty years, he reiterated how harmonious relationships were between communities. I decided I had better stop asking what everyone seemed to suggest was a stupid question. Perhaps I had misunderstood where PraiseMoves was coming from.

I looked at the six shrines around the room, noticing the yoni bowl set erotically next to a phallic stone – apparently Mondays were the day for pouring milk on Shiva's lingam. I spotted, too, the fresh pear left at one of the shrines, just like Catherine's pomegranates, and as a man came in and stood reverently at one of the shrines I recognised Mountain pose. Peterborough, where I'd come because of a resistance by one faith to another, was teaching me the interconnections between spiritual traditions. As I stood rather wide-eyed in the middle of the idols and chrysanthemum heads and nightclub-style LED lights flashing around the shrines, the mandir's openness was evident. It wasn't only a matter of the easy welcome to me who clearly came from a very different tradition, but in the signs on the noticeboard advertising a 'spiritual congregation on the life and philosophy of Sree Sree Thakur Anukulchandra' where 'everyone across community, faith and race is invited'.

My guide took time to explain to me the different gods (those 'gods, little "G."' that Laurette had identified as 'the real danger') represented round the room. I had never thought much before about the Hindu or any other pantheon, beyond a general incredulity that these pale dolls could be believed to be any kind of deity. Perhaps I had been closer to Dr Willis than I realised. But as I was introduced in turn to Rama and Parvati and Ganesh I thought of my process of selection for my yoga sessions depending on what I feel I most importantly need that day. 'Yoga for self-confidence', 'yoga for patience', 'yoga for flexibility'. We choose which narrative we're going to need on any given day, and so it suddenly seemed logical that you might need help with love one day; help from the Lawgiver the next.

I asked about yoga's relationship to Hinduism. 'It is part of our culture, but not of our religion,' I was told. And watching the *bindi* mark being placed carefully by a worshipper on the 'third eye' and having it explained to me that 'we make the bindi mark at the point of our third eye, which is where we focus when we meditate', just as I'd been told about at my yoga session in London, the heritage started to make more sense.

A service was about to start so I stopped asking questions and moved from learning *about* to learning *by*. All I had to do was to sit but it was hot, and incense started to swirl and I started feeling queasy in the waves of unfamiliar sounds and scents and sense. A quavering singing had started up in the small congregation of half a dozen people and it went on and on. But when the 'Gayatri mantra' began and I heard its first word, *om*, I was back on familiar ground.

I had been doing Peterborough wrong to think it was defined by Dr Laurette Willis. Even at the church where her PraiseMoves was practised, the welcome was palpable. When I got there I was taken on a brief tour by the petite, practical and enthusiastic leader, Ronna, who's from Malaysia and was brought up Buddhist. She said that fifty languages were spoken at the church.

She told me briefly how she had come to be 'saved', and I was struck as I had been at the temple by the openness of the faithful, by the lack of embarrassment in talking about deeply personal experiences and beliefs that most people I knew could only discuss with a scattergun of inverted commas – like those I just put around 'saved'.

She took me to see the enormous auditorium capable of hosting this world congregation, with a gleaming drum set on the stage. Thankfully for my performance anxiety, this was not where we would be practising PraiseMoves; our session was held in a sleek conference room.

We started with a prayer where Ronna thanked God for bringing me and the other woman attending for the first time, and for our fellowship in a broken world. And then she turned on the introductory video. One of my good friends is a wonderful wise and intuitive American Christian whom I'd told about my plan to come to PraiseMoves. 'Ohh, I hope it's not too cheesy,' she'd said. Her familiarity with the genre had forewarned her for what I had no idea of.

At the beginning we were shown footage on the big screen at the front where Laurette appeared, many times life-size. She took us through some warm-up moves, poised at the head of a V-shape made up of people standing on a stepped stage. She told us that this programme had the potential for change in us. The woman next to me muttered 'Yes. Change, Amen.' I felt very self-conscious.

Laurette was in her sixties and well-preserved with an iron perkiness I found irritating, if not sinister. She had a touch of Aunt Sarah from *The Handmaid's Tale*.

But Ronna was with us, interpreting below the huge display of Laurette somewhere far away from Peterborough. And Ronna was human, friendly, listening, encouraging. The others were welcoming too, even when I explained, in answer to their curious questions, that I was not a believer, just here to try it out.

We were all women, though Ronna said that there were some men who wanted to join but not all the ladies were happy to have men there. 'Last week there was a pose like childbirth.' My Handmaid's antennae were quivering.

Then Laurette took us through a routine where we mimed putting on the armour of God: the breastplate of righteousness, and the helmet of salvation, and being shod with the gospel of peace. Now, she said, we were ready for our day. She led us on a 'Jericho march' (on the spot). My American friend was wiser than I had ever known.

I was trying to get the divine light in me to salute the divine light in Laurette, and I was finding it difficult. Just when I'd found a way to admire her – her courage, perhaps, her conviction, the fact that she was doing something about sharing what she believed in, unlike so many people in the 'whatever' world – she'd do something like suggest we smile which would prompt her to sing out a little off-script comment like 'because a cheerful heart doeth good like a medicine, Proverbs seventeen twenty-two' and I would grind my teeth again.

She reminded us, too, that if we did manage to get stronger by doing all this exercise then the glory belonged to God.

And if we injured ourselves? If we found that we were weaker than we thought, older, more fragile? I was pretty sure no-one here would be laying such eventualities at God's door.

It wasn't always easy to follow Laurette on the video because she was wearing unrevealing clothing that I assumed was making a point about modesty, following a spate of media coverage of yoga pants and their sweatily close relationship to nudity, male desire and female responsibility for these things. However, the dark baggy trousers she'd chosen to wear instead didn't make it easy to see exactly how she was positioning herself. This was, no doubt, the precise aim of modesty in dress, but the opposite of what is needed for a physical-training video. Perhaps we could have used small porcelain mannequins like Victorians used to demonstrate pain in unmentionable places.

Ronna then led us into our poses. They had names that were new to me, and some of them were new poses too. Each pose was linked with a verse from scripture and as we held the pose we recited the text together along with the chapter and verse reference too. I had thought I would resist this, feeling hypocritical, but in most cases the verses were reminders of the poetry in the Bible, the forms of words worn familiar by generations of tongues. 'They that wait upon the Lord shall renew their strength; they shall mount up with wings as eagles; they shall run, and not be weary; and they shall walk, and not faint. Isaiah 40:31,' we repeated with ascending fervour as we held Eagle pose.

Into Tree pose ('He shall be like a tree planted by the rivers of water, that brings forth its fruit in its season, whose leaf also shall not wither; and whatever he does shall prosper. Psalm 1:3') and the pose that I will always now call Mustard-seed, the curled-up ball formed by drawing in your knees to your chest as you lie on your back. ('If you have faith as a mustard seed, you can say to this mulberry tree, "Be pulled up by the roots and be planted in the sea" and it would obey you. Luke 17:6').

It was an inspiring reminder of the centrality of faith; the glorious certainty of the saved. There were no such certainties in my usual yoga routines. There were references to human frailty and untapped human power, but no easy answers. Ronna's faith seemed to be built on the idea of an easy answer being available. If you could – just – have faith. It wasn't a certainty I was used to experiencing, and trying it out for just a few moments in a conference room near the Tesco on the outskirts of Peterborough felt comforting. I distrusted that comfort though, with every rational bone in my quaveringly physical body. I was reminded, however, of the closest I had come to experiencing it before, just a year previously when I had a violent and poorly-timed attack of food poisoning. Poorly timed because it came over a day when I was travelling, and I had the distinction of throwing up in three countries in one day – an early-morning airport, a transfer airport, and finally back in London. As the illness moved into its thirty-sixth hour and my dehydration, weakness and disorientation peaked, I felt wretched (as well as retched). I was travelling alone, and too scared to let on to airline staff or fellow travellers of how bad I was feeling in case I was denied onward travel. Doubled up over my seatbelt I was terrifyingly aware of myself as a tiny speck (now I would say a mustard seed) flung through the air, with only the dubious machinery of a small Air Serbia aeroplane to hold me. And then I had a vision of a huge hand stretched out under our plane, fingers curling beneath me and all on board; the universe cradling me. 'You have hedged me behind and before, and laid Your hand upon me. Psalm 139:5,' we recited.

We moved on to more Psalms – 'I raise my eyes to the hills from whence cometh my help,' we called out, standing in a quad stretch with one arm raised as if hailing the power of the natural world. This was followed by 'He will not suffer thy foot to be moved: he that keepeth thee will not slumber,' – a risky thing to claim as we were all wobbling.

'Beautiful shape; well done Elizabeth,' Ronna called out to me by name as I bent back into what I would call Bow pose. My chest would have swelled – if the pose would have allowed it.

'By the rivers of Babylon, there we sat down, yea, we wept when we remembered Zion. We hung our harps upon the willows in the midst of it. Psalm 137:1–2,' had me and the older lady on the mat next to me humming Boney M (the others were too young to know what had set us off) as we wept into a bent-over Tree pose.

A particularly complicated pose brought us with the soles of our feet together as in Cobbler but lifted like in Boat pose. We then threaded our arms under our legs to come out the other side, by our feet. As we did so we were invited to repeat 'The flowers appear on the earth; the time of the singing of birds is come, and the voice of the turtle is heard in our land; Solomon 2:12'. We were all a little strangled with our chests compressed by the combined tension of all our contorted limbs. Definitely more 'voice of the turtle' than 'singing of birds'.

It was nice to have these texts to think about while holding a particularly uncomfortable stretch, but this was the fundamental, fundamentalist, difference between yoga and PraiseMoves. Ronna referenced it at the beginning of the class: that in yoga, people seek to empty their mind while in PraiseMoves they seek to fill their mind – with the word of God. Christians are people of the Word and the Book and so perhaps it makes sense to do whatever can be done to multiply the Words you have in your head. But for myself, there are quite enough words in there. My meditation and yoga sessions are the times when I still those words and allow in the silence, interrupted only by the rush of breath in and out. One of the techniques I'd been using to help my meditation recently, and to manage the words that came unbidden when I was trying to focus, had been imagining how I would deal with them if they were spoken aloud by me in a church or yoga session or library, or any contemplative silent place. Suddenly, the 'do I have enough bread left for a sandwich this evening?' or 'did I look stupid when I asked that question in the meeting?' and 'oh, it was so good to be held in Rob's arms this morning' were not just lapses in concentration but revealed for the ludicrous or inappropriate or trivial interruptions they were. 'Shh,' said another, deeper, inner voice when they started up; she was something between a vestal virgin and a school prefect, 'please be quiet; we're trying to meditate.' And for a while at least the voices would be quiet and the words would go away.

Here, the vestal prefect would have no chance.

I was reminded by what political prisoners in Enver Hoxha's Albania had told me about their incarceration. One of those I'd spoken to was in prison only for owning a Bob Dylan record. He said that the worst thing was the endless reading out loud of Enver Hoxha's works, so that at all times of day you couldn't think your own thoughts. Laurette was a long way from Enver Hoxha, but I couldn't help thinking that her beliefs and fears about the fundamental nature of human beings and what would happen to a mind left unattended might not be so different.

Not only did I believe, ever more passionately, that silences were good for me, but my instinct was that if there was something greater than me – 'the Absolute' – then my best way to communicate with It was to allow this space. As Rumi says:

> Make of yourself a blank page, a piece of empty ground
> where a seed may be planted by the Absolute.

I felt that if I spent my time learning the seed catalogue by heart then there would be no space for the Absolute to do the planting of any of it.

At the end of the session we were invited to lie down, as you would move into Shavasana at the end of a yoga session. But where I was used to this being a time of absorption and of reflection, here we had Aunt Laurette reading gospel to us from the big screen.

Afterwards, Ronna organised our group into a circle, holding hands. She led us in prayer which I found unexpectedly moving. As well as giving general thanks, she specifically asked God to bless me, reminding me that God made our tongues to speak truth and asking for us to be agents of healing in a broken world. It made me wonder whether my Aunt Sarah comment had been quite fair.

After the class, while I waited for my taxi to the station, Ronna and three of her friends who'd been at the class sat with me. One woman was from Hong Kong and gave her story of how she was saved, while going through a divorce. Another in the class had had a strong African accent, while the woman who'd hummed with me to Boney M had been white. For all the cathedral's welcome notices I'd seen no such diversity there. As one of the Malaysian women got out decaf Malaysian coffee and tasty butter-free sponge cakes and shared it with me in a humble little communion, I felt I had misunderstood the redemptive power of human beings, of all backgrounds and beliefs, when they come together in a community. This was what faith – perhaps any faith – could achieve, and I had not even had as much as a mustard seed.

Gratitude diary entry
my hand-crocheted top bought at a Balkan market stall

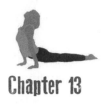

Chapter 13

Kundalini – Awakening the Coiled Serpents of The Cotswolds

*'Exhale, focusing on your left eye, then your right eye and
then the tip of the nose, and thinking wa hey guru'*

The body was lithe as Lycra and, with a ripple, it curled round itself
to rest its head nonchalantly on its rear end in an impossible twist.

I was in the snake house of the Cotswold Wildlife Park and
Gardens, which has one of the largest reptile collections in the UK. I
was here as research and preparation for my Cotswold class of yoga
named for *kundalini*, 'the coiled one'.

The Kundalini yoga I'd encountered at the dog yoga session
offers physical practices and meditation targeting this coiled 'snake'
of energy, visualised as residing at the base of the spine. So here I was
on the outskirts of Burford gazing at a green tree python who had
fixed me with a yogic stare. In the next enclosure was a puff adder,
whose sign told us it was this species which causes more human
fatalities than almost any other. I would be going into the Kundalini
session with a fitting fear for what I might be awakening, with these
signboards echoing in my head along with the harrowing accounts of
the orgasmic experiences of those who had released their kundalini.

I was taking my mother, a fit woman in her sixties but one who
had very little yoga experience. In the past forty-four years, since my
own birth brought an end to her antenatal yoga classes, she had done
yoga only twice, when I'd taken her along to classes.

'I've googled what to wear,' she told me when we had met at the train station. 'Because we're going to be entering a sacred space you're invited to wear clothes that set your practice apart from your street clothes.'

I had changed into leggings and a stretchy top in the unsacred space of the train toilet. I thought of the Peterborough mandir and wondered about what sacred spaces gained by making people feel dirty on entering them.

I smiled indulgently at my mother, pretending to more expertise than I had. It's true that I had practised more yoga than her, but my experience of Kundalini was little more advanced than hers. I had taken a class some years previously but I hadn't gone back because I had found it faintly unsettling, and it hadn't given me the feeling of a reconnected body that I'd had from other yoga experiences. I remembered the jerking of the exercises (which was designed to release and direct the flow of kundalini energy from the lower centres to the higher energetic centres) and something I thought had been called 'Breast of Fire' – a panting breathing technique which had indeed left lactic acid around my middle.

I'd been taught by a French speaker then and only later realised this was 'Brea*th* of Fire' wiz exotic pronunciation.

But perhaps the most powerfully unsettling of the exercises or *kriyas* we'd done in the accented class I'd attended was where we were invited to call out 'ma' to the world mother as we repeated a jerking movement over our outstretched leg. The semi-dark room was filled with the puffing and bleating of what sounded like lost children, my own wailing voice among them. I'd been sixteen hundred miles away from my mother at the time, and I'd found it an unexpectedly moving experience calling out her name like a baby.

And now here she was, summoned by my call! And we left the snakes to attend to the serpents we carried around with us.

In fact my mother had come to meet me from her home in a small Cotswold village which has a particular and unexpectedly significant role in the history of yoga in Britain. In 1732 the Oxfordshire village of Churchill was the birthplace of one Warren Hastings. My mother was involved with the village's Heritage Centre whose exhibition was where I'd learned about Hastings's life and achievements. Despite having been born into a poor family and going out to India as a clerk with the British East India Company, Hastings soon built a reputation there for hard work which eventually led to him becoming the first governor-general of India. It was this Cotswold boy who determined that Hindus would be judged according to Hindu law rather than British common law. As Indologist David Gordon White explains, since Hindu law was written in the ancient language of Sanskrit, 'an unanticipated consequence of the British occupation of Bengal was the urgent necessity to learn Sanskrit'.

With the commercial incentive of litigation, Britons begin to learn Sanskrit and to publish the necessary dictionaries. And it was not long before hobbyists, younger brothers and spiritually-minded traders started using the new tools and knowledge to discover the fifth-century yoga sutras. And so it was that the Cotswolds opened up a channel that led from Bengal to Edinburgh's Lululemon, to HM Prison Downview, and to our destination this evening, the 'Inner Temple' yoga studio.

This was on the outskirts of Cirencester and I imagined it would be the kind of place where women would turn up with their yoga mats propped in straw baskets 'like baguettes in a black-and-white photograph from France' as *Yoga Bitch* writer Suzanne Morrison describes it. The class was led by Karen who gave us a smiling welcome, remembering our names from the email booking.

The centre seemed to be a converted chapel, an old stone building with a small foyer area and a studio space in low light. The foyer was all Cotswolds – homemade plum jam for sale and handcrafted lavender eye masks for use in Shavasana. Inside were ten practitioners – all female bar one – settling on their yoga mats and zafu cushions.

The beginning was chatty; Karen had been away on holiday and asked some questions about the sound bath she'd missed. I looked up at this conversation about enfolding yourself in sound vibrations, and inner transformation through resonation; I was hoping I'd have a chance to try it one day myself.

Gently, Karen moved from the general conversation to a structured round where she asked everyone to introduce themselves by name and one word about how they were feeling. It gave my mother the chance to blurt out 'nervous', and for me to mention my travels and the feeling today of having 'landed'. We checked in our baggage as people described themselves as 'fine' or 'stressed' or 'exhausted'. One woman had just received a speeding ticket.

It also grounded the practice in the realities of our days, and of modern life, outside the 'Inner Temple.' It's one thing to talk about peace and nourishing breath and relaxation, and another to have a conversation with a traffic warden.

Already Karen had started weaving us into a supportive group, and when Rachel panicked that she might have left her car lights on it seemed natural that we should all wait until she'd popped out to check them.

We began with seven minutes – *seven minutes* – of *pranayama* breathing techniques, inhaling for a count of five, holding the breath for a count of five and then releasing it for a count of five.

We moved on to some chanting of *om* and then before we started a physical practice Karen talked a bit about current issues, particularly the aggression and chaos she said we could feel at the moment with Mars so near.

The physical practice began with a Sufi Grind, sitting cross-legged with our palms cupping our kneecaps to anchor us as we rotated our torso in wide circles. It gave a deep massage and she reminded us that this is how atoms and planets move, and that by joining it we made ourselves part of this universal movement. She also quoted Joseph Pilates: 'You are only as young as your spine is flexible.'

I knew it would be coming, and now Karen announced Breath (I still heard it in my head as *breast*) of Fire. She told us to put our hands up in a V shape high above our head and then we activated our abdominal muscles as if we were being punched repeatedly and rhythmically in the stomach. Slightly faster than once per second we contracted the muscles to expel air in a desperate-sounding panting. 'Don't worry about the inhalation; that will happen naturally once you've forced the air out,' she said and it was true that your body gasps back what has been so rudely pushed out of it. It was a curious intimacy in a small dimly-lit room with these strangers – and my mother – to hear the kind of noises you usually don't hear from another human until you've been dating for a while. I don't know how long we kept this up because it felt like hours but it must have been at least five minutes. I wasn't sure what that green tree python coiled around my coccyx was making of this but I certainly couldn't believe it could sleep through it.

Next we used the breath of fire to accompany a repeated Frog. Squatting with heels up and fingertips on the floor we pushed bums in the air and straightened our legs before returning to the squat.

After a block of these we moved into Cow, leg up in the air, and then Cat where we repeatedly punched a fist straight out ('and through all the crap in our lives', said Karen). We sat in Hero pose and then put our forehead on the floor while clapping our hands once behind us, bouncing back up again until I felt dizzy; we repeated a routine where we flapped our fingers and then pulled our arms back sharply, bringing our elbows to touch an acupressure point on the rib cage.

This is typical of Kundalini yoga's approach which applies pressure to points and meridians on the body. I don't understand these meridians but I believe in a wiring system of some kind which dissected bodies don't reveal – I know that applying pressure on the bottom point of the V formed by my thumb and forefinger turns off my headaches as if it were a switch. And having discovered the quirk or kink in my body which gave me a gentle but distinct pain in the outside of my right thigh on a certain day every month, it was in my Kundalini yoga session that I'd discovered that this point on the upper leg is linked to the reproductive organs.

So although all this was bewildering I was open to it doing some good. It certainly must have woken anything cowering anywhere in my being, but I couldn't honestly say that I could identify any physical benefit in my jolted body. However, the next stage of the class was transformational, whatever my inner puff adder may have thought of it. Karen led us through a practical process to bring about peace.

As we inhaled we had to think of a situation of conflict. Easy – I had been in a heated argument before the weekend where I'd felt disrespected and had sensed the impact on a friend of mine who'd been with me. I'd tried to manage the situation and had both said too much and not said enough. I could still boil to think of it.

Step two: exhale, focusing as you do so on your left eye, then right eye, then the tip of your nose as you think 'wa hey guru' (no, I don't know why. It translates just as you would from the Geordie – a teacher's greeting). Next we had to relive the conflict, remembering the details of how we felt. And we exhaled, focusing again on left eye, right eye and then the tip of the nose, *wa hey guru*. On the next inhalation we had to play out the situation again, thinking of it from the point of view of the other person. Exhale as before. On the subsequent inhalation we had to forgive that person, and forgive ourselves for our anger and our part in it. Repeat the previous exhalation. On the final inhalation we were invited to let it all go into the universe, before exhaling again.

It was transformational. Try it! Taking a situation that had made me see red at the time but also had raised my heartbeat and hackles every time I'd remembered it in the four or five days since it happened, I finally made my peace with it.

The next day I sent a message to the friend who'd been with me when I'd got so angry, and who'd been equally furious at what we'd faced together. I told her enthusiastically of my epiphany, of how the other guy might have felt, now I'd seen the incident from his point of view, eager to share what I'd learned and the journey I'd been on, in just five in-breaths.

Her reply was scathing: 'He is old enough to understand at least what respect is.'

Which shows that you can't fast-forward these processes. I was sure she would have got to the point I had if she'd sat through the rest of our Kundalini session. Did you really need to do the focus on the left eye, right eye, tip of nose (*wa hey guru*)? Whether out of embarrassment or efficiency I'd missed that out of my message.

After our peace-building there was more chanting. We ended with our hands in Prayer pose at the chakra above the head, then brought to the second chakra, at the 'third eye' and then to our heart, representing 'right seeing,' 'right thinking,' and 'right speaking' before bowing to the floor – 'heads lower than hearts' – a more comfortable metaphor than it was a position. Out of the corner of my eye I saw my mother bowing confidently.

Afterwards I asked some of the other women how the Kundalini practice helped them. One was wearing a T-shirt with 'sat nam' in big block letters. I knew this was the Kundalini phrase translating as something like 'true identity' – a neat substitution on a T-shirt where you might normally see the 'assumed identities' of a brand name. She coloured at my compliment on the shirt – 'I printed it myself!' – and yes, the weekly Kundalini practice was an important part of her life, 'but I struggle to keep it going away from the studio.'

Another woman overheard the conversation, 'I don't know why we do it but when you feel the effect then you stop caring about why.'

My Cotswold yoga journey wasn't over with the end of the Kundalini class as I had a yogic train to catch to get back to London. 'Yogic' because of the rather unlikely pairing of Chiltern Railways with the University of Oxford Mindfulness Centre, which had resulted in a leaflet of 'train yoga moves' offered to commuters to 'promote mindfulness'. A statement had referenced the railway company's partnership with a mental health charity for their year's fundraising and their hope to leave their passengers 're-energised' (with a short *yama* at the end, requesting that 'passengers remember to keep their feet off the seats when attempting the poses').

The seated poses had non-Sanskrit names like Choo-choo (a breathing exercise), the Onward Journey neck stretch and Ticket

Inspection holding the arms as they usually are in Eagle. My train was not a commuter service and I had plenty of space and not much audience so I even ventured a Tree pose when the train was at a stop. However, I wasn't sure that I felt truly 're-energised' by Chiltern's recommendations. The true release was in letting go of everything dredged up by that argument. Imagine if every commuter on Chiltern Railways instead followed those 'ten steps to peace' as part of their journey home.

Gratitude diary entry
Rob kissing my neck

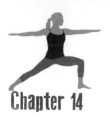

Chapter 14

Britain's Noisiest City – a Sound Bath in Newcastle

'There's an energy vortex in the centre of my shed'

I wanted to swim through sound! I wanted sound to swim through me! Following up the enthusiasm of the Cirencester yoginis about their sound baths, I knew I wanted to try one.

And the place to take one would surely be Britain's noisiest city. According to my online research, that honour goes to Newcastle, so I booked in for a resonant experience somewhere loud along the Tyne.

In the train on the way up I wondered what it meant to say that Newcastle was Britain's noisiest city. How would I tell? I couldn't imagine there would be some immediate barrage of sound on the opening of the train door.

It was therefore something of a surprise to disembark into the airy space beneath Newcastle Central's Victorian arches and to be greeted by a 24-piece orchestra playing 'Can't Take My Eyes Off You' with gusto.

Street Orchestra Live are apparently a 'pop-up' orchestra and they play across the country so it was pure chance that this was my introduction to Newcastle's soundtrack, but it was a good way to sensitise my ears.

And there was plenty to sensitise them. There were buskers at what seemed like every opportunity (later in the day as I came up the escalator from the Metro the little girl ahead of me took in the guy with his guitar standing at the top and asked wearily of her father 'why is there *always* someone playing music?' – I 'heard' her). On the bus, a group of young men were singing. Later, on the train, a group of women were singing; everywhere I went, Newcastle was in full voice.

Along with this music was an extraordinary amount of dancing. Granted, I was in town on a summer weekend, prime time for hen do's, and England had just made World Cup progress unprecedented in my lifetime, but there was literally dancing in the streets. Not just ironic drunken capering, self-conscious shuffling, or people swaying as what they actually tried to do was to stand up while under the influence. I saw those things, but I also saw expert, careful, beautiful full-on dancing because you know, sometimes the rhythm just gets you. It was unlike anything I'd seen outside of Cuba.

But the drunken capering… At times the city looked like a Hogarth print. As I walked through the city centre, pub doors burst open to grey-faced young men staggering out. Sorrowful young women crouched in painful shoes and were quietly sick; older women (also in painful shoes) swore and lunged at each other; men called out incoherently, brayed and sprayed with laughter.

Official statistics suggest this was not an unrepresentative experience – the city has identified the need for a 'strategy for reducing the harm caused by alcohol to individuals, families and communities'. Called *Safe, Sensible and Social*, its plan begins with alarming data on the scope of Newcastle's drink problem. Newcastle has one of the highest rates of binge drinking in England, with about thirty per cent of adults estimated to binge drink. Alcohol-related hospital admissions, chronic liver disease and alcohol-related deaths are all higher in Newcastle than the average for both the northeast and England. Alcohol-related hospital stays by residents of

Newcastle are approximately seventy per cent higher than England's average. Newcastle and Sunderland's women have also been given more on-the-spot fines for nuisance public drinking than women in any other region.

Escaping these perils of the city centre I made my way to Wallsend station, the stop for my gong bath. At the station there were two young teenage girls, one blonde, one Asian, sitting spitting at the platform, each cradling a bottle like a baby. On the other platform, across the tracks, sat others of their age. Occasionally someone would dart across the track. In between, the kids called across the rails to one another, 'What youse doing?' It was a bleak picture of boredom and risky behaviours feeding off one another.

In the nineteenth century this area was called 'the jakes of Newcastle' and the station certainly stank of urine. I set off quickly for my Airbnb – the cheapest room I'd been able to find. It was in a house run by a woman whose profile described her as a former teacher who lived alone. Her home sounded like a refuge from the intoxicated celebrations outside and I knocked gratefully at the front door.

I got no answer. Having checked I was in the right place I tried again with greater confidence, and not a little desperation. There was another silence, and then the sound of someone lurching to the door. She opened it to me and stood rocking in confusion while I came to terms with the fact that this might not be the refuge I had hoped. Once she finally focused on me she remembered my name from the Airbnb booking and led me in and teetered up the stairs to show me my room. Slurringly she said she'd like to have a *lrong llrrong* chat with me but I begged tiredness after my travels.

I locked the bedroom door and got into bed. All seemed quiet except for occasional passers-by singly or in groups wailing football songs with the incomprehensibility of mantras that have been oft repeated. *Fu ballskum inome*. They intoned them wonderingly in the same way that I'd found that chants in my yoga classes simultaneously lost all meaning and gained a deeper meaning the more times you said them.

An hour or so later there was a banging on my bedroom door and my Airbnb hostess – the one who had escorted me up here only a short while previously – demanded half-afraid, half-belligerent, and entirely drunk, to know who was there.

With a mixture of irritation, indulgence and fear I called out my name and she retreated muttering an uncertain 'good night then; sleep well'.

I did not.

The next morning I left promptly to explore Wallsend. This, I was prepared to bet, was not currently the noisiest place in Britain. With a name derived from its being the point where a now defunct archaeological structure had run out, perhaps it did not attract go-getters. And on a Sunday morning it was a place of cats and Christians and care workers changing shift; a place with the self-sufficient quiet of people with dogs or people who jog. I wandered the streets, past the Segedunum fort which had defended the end of Hadrian's Wall. The wall itself was mainly evidenced now by stumpy stones like the gap-teethed remnants of a big smile, but the remains of buildings could be seen. The settlement had been a Roman garrison for around three hundred years, up to AD400. With 120 cavalry and 480 infantry stationed there I tried to imagine the sounds I could have heard back then – the reverberations that could have been absorbed by this wall. Calls in Latin – and pig Latin; the calls of pigs. The noise of 120 horses, and of 600 men – the sound of their orders, their arguments, their dice games and laughter. I imagined some of the lasses I'd seen last night, probably still in uncomfortable shoes, but these with leather thongs; I imagined the local voices calling out to soldiers they had as husbands, lovers, customers. And the military sounds of war-readiness – metal on stone, beat on drum. And the buskers (and maybe also the children still asking 'why is there *always* someone playing music?') with simple exotic instruments singing out songs from across the Empire.

Over a millennium later, collieries were sunk here and there would have been other sounds. Hammer on rock, trundling wheels, explosions.

Now all silent.

There was a shopping centre whose marketing team had smartly named it The Forum, but which was as deserted as Segedunum.

The train station had been proud of the neighbourhood's Roman connection – it had trumpeted that it was the only station in the world with Latin and English signage, though I couldn't imagine the 'what youse doing?' kids last night staring with anything other than incomprehension at the *'noli fumare'* signs accompanied by the line through a cigarette on *'Suggestus* (platform) i'.

I continued past Poundland and pawnshops, nail bars and wine bars, all closed in the early morning of course, but also past places permanently closed. There was the Citizens Advice Bureau and charity shops and churches… an index of poverty, and the ways out and the ways to make it bearable while you're in. And then there were the fitness centres. There was a boxing hall and a dance studio and a gym, and then finally I came to the Vault.

This was where my 'bath' was to be held but it was not until the evening, so now I had found it, I had a day ahead of me to explore Newcastle. I took the Metro back into town, listening all the while.

I sensed the city's sore head this morning, and even into afternoon. But there were still things to hear; the distinctive sounds of a distinctive town: the cry of gulls overhead, the way mouths formed their words. I really was called 'pet' and even young women used the word 'lass'. The garage I passed had a proud sign on it proclaiming 'We're shut; we've gone yem' and there were restaurants with names like 'The Toon'. The bus I saw going through town had 'Gannin' alang the Scotswood Road to see the Blaydon Races' blazoned on the side and another bus company sign, knowing it would be understood by all those it was really speaking to, assured its public they were getting 'a canny good deal'.

There were distinctive behaviours, too, that you wouldn't see in the south. As I stood frowning over a map a man asked whether I was lost and directed me to where I needed to go. Twice (once on entering a Metro train compartment and once going into a shop) men invited me to enter ahead of them, and insisted when I demurred.

The differences made me feel uncomfortable. Listening out, I was even more aware of it in my voice. I was Not From Round Here (I heard myself say it with the vowels all long, all wrong). I had always been on the winning side; I was indulged, over-resourced, privileged. The people I was speaking to didn't seem to mind, but I did. I couldn't even talk about the place without feeling self-conscious. New*castle* to rhyme with 'hassle' (as the local people would say it, but did it sound like I was taking the mickey?) or New*castle* to rhyme with 'parcel' (the way I would talk about any other 'castle', but marking me out immediately)?

These differences were current, but they were also historical. On the Metro I learned that my ticket could take me to Jarrow. I hadn't realised we were so near a name which meant nothing to me but flat caps and rainy streets and tough, undaunted men with black-and-white – and grey – faces 'marching on London'.

Their spirit was kept alive in the centre of Newcastle too, where the Grey's Monument at the heart of the city had been decked out in banners to make what was being called a 'Workers' Maypole'. The banners each articulated one of the aspirations of the Labour movement – 'Leisure for All', 'Eight Hour Working Day' – making a multicoloured stick of seaside rock out of the monument dedicated to a man I only knew as a bergamot tea. I was Not From Round Here… Only later did I research how Earl Grey deserved his monument, and more, for the passing of the 1832 Great Reform Act.

There were other, less obvious, pieces of public art for those who were learning to look: along Grainger Street I found a small bronze plaque fixed into the ground:

> Nathan Walker walked past here 47 times during 1968
> on the 21st May 1968 he looked up

Once I was online I googled Nathan Walker and his 1968 epiphany but it was only with a bit of hunting through the twilight world of geocacher forums that I found him. Or rather I found what he represented. This was one of four 'antiplaques' set up in the street to celebrate ordinary people's everyday experiences. Others apparently read 'Mrs Mary Howard adjusted her hat in the reflection in this window 3rd June, 1921', 'David Williams watched the rain from here 7th September, 1979', and 'Ann Huxtable waited here for a friend who did not arrive 8th December, 1952'.

Further on, in my careful, mindful, meditative walk through town (whose other purpose, by the way, was to find another Primark to get some new leggings for the next yoga session) I found words carved into the granite kerbstone, one letter per quoin. The spacing of the letters forced you to walk along sounding them out like a primary school child.

'F-R-O-M H-E-R-E I-T I-S 9-2-5-9-C-M (H-O-W A-R-E Y-O-U F-E-E-L-I-N-G?) T-O H-E-R-E'. It was a cute way to slow people down as they moved around the shopping streets.

Later, subjecting the town to my ongoing auscultation, I found in a mall part of the 'Sound of a City' *Whistle* installation. A board explained it:

> Once upon a time the North was alive with the sound of steam engines, and to remind us how important the North was to engineering and the railways, artist Steve Messam has created this spectacular sound installation. At 1pm every day, a series of steam engine whistles will cascade around Newcastle's ancient town walls, completing the two-mile circuit in under 30 seconds.

Next to the board stood a tall pole with a brass dome contraption on the top, which I guessed could be noisy. Newcastle was working hard for its decibels.

I was ready for the calming effect I had been promised from a sound bath and travelled back to Wallsend's Vault. I was early and the group before me were still on a shamanic journey. They welcomed me graciously – especially gracious since my knock on the door interrupted their travels through what they were calling Middle Earth – and I sat in an anteroom as unobtrusively as possible and tried to work on my laptop until their session could finish. Threads of their conversation made it through the door – whether to get on the Peace Pipe mailing list or to set up a chanting Facebook page, the role of fairies in 'soul retrieval' for people who are suicidal. One woman told the others 'there's an energy vortex in the centre of my shed'.

'Really?' There was perhaps understandable skepticism.

'Well, yes, I've created it with amethyst and rose crystals.'

I tried not to listen in, and kept myself busy with looking at the literature that had been left at the centre advertising various services, like Trevor, the spiritual clairvoyant ('gives proof of life everlasting; party bookings welcome').

When the group had dispersed I got talking to Christine who would be leading our sound bath. She's a yoga teacher and runs a youth group as well as a chanting group and leads shamanic journeys in courses and workshops from Newcastle to Glastonbury – so there was plenty to talk about.

Shortly afterwards, Catherine arrived to join the sound bath, here for her third time. She told me that she did Kundalini yoga at The Vault which is how she'd heard about the sound baths and had started to attend these too. She said there were usually at least half a dozen people, but that in a larger group people didn't seem as open to talking to each other. After a short wait we concluded that this would be the sum of our group today and we all badly wanted our little group to gel, to multiply our energy. We discussed our names; Christine's middle name is Elizabeth and my middle name is Katherine; my mother's name is Christine.

Catherine said in a small voice that her middle name was Louise.

But when we talked more, Catherine described her work in marketing for a local shipping company, and her hope of finding a social enterprise where she could share her skills; I shared the need

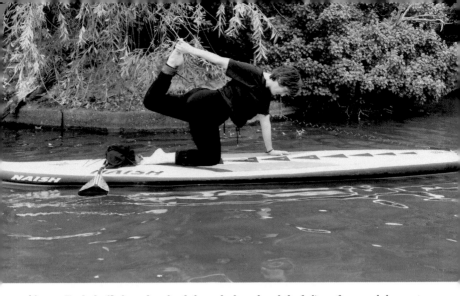

Above: *Each shuffle brought a lurch from the board and the feeling of a surge below me; every action a reaction*
Stand-Up Paddleboard yoga on a lake in Nottingham (CP)

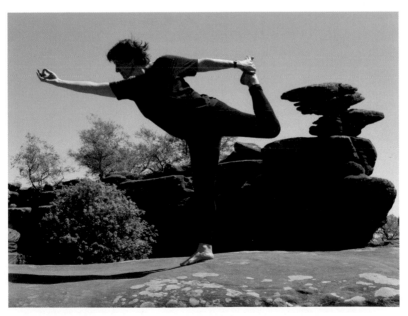

Above: *Where Yorkshire grit meets mindfulness*
Yoga with the National Trust at Brimham Rocks, North Yorkshire (PM)

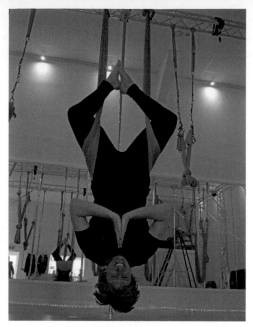

Above: *A tussle with gravity*
Aerial yoga in Godalming (CG)

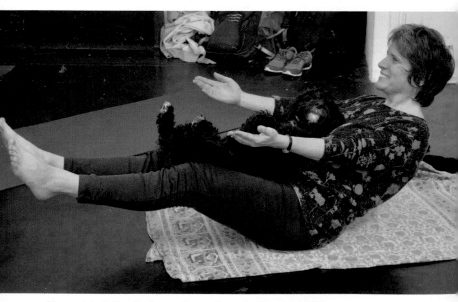

Above: *Ms Crikey Barker teaches me Doga in Shoreditch* (JR)

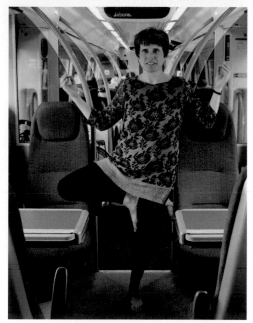

Above: *Travelling with Chiltern Trains who recently produced a leaflet of 'train yoga moves'* (EG)

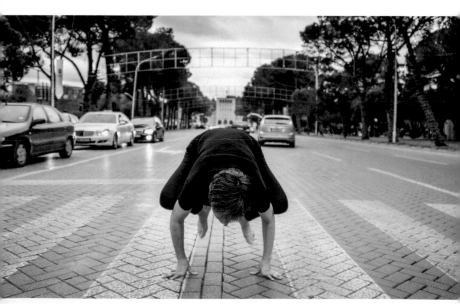

Above: *It was so obvious that falling onto my skull was what I was most likely to do* Managing Crow pose at last (EVL)

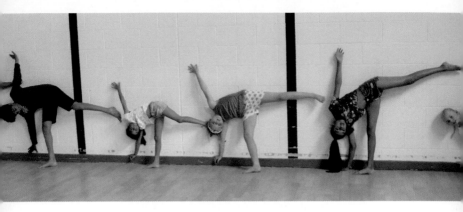

Above: *Some friends think it's cool; some think it's weird*
Children's yoga in Slough (EG)

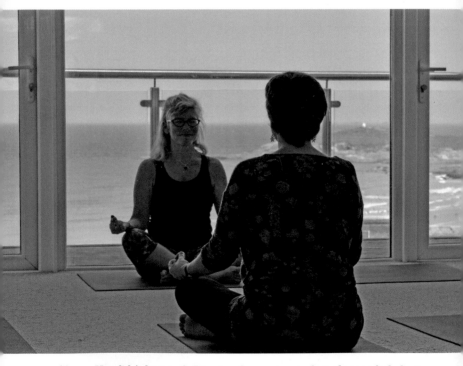

Above: *You didn't have to do Lion pose for your jaw to drop: the room looked out over the length of Fistral Bay where the legendary surf was drawing in and out with a reassuring ujjayi breath*
Yin yoga at Oceanflow yoga studio in Newquay (CF)

for the social enterprise I ran in the Balkans to have greater marketing expertise. It was, we agreed, meant to be.

And in a way it was. In another way it was just three odd women looking for purpose on a Sunday evening in the town where the wall runs out.

The 'bathing' Christine offers is metaphorical only, so there would be no liquids and we would stay fully dressed, and we were invited to settle ourselves lying comfortably on our mats while Christine gave a brief introduction. She started with references to the broken world we live in – and reminded me of Ronna.

She invited us to take deep breaths and with each out-breath to let go of what no longer served us. Then she started to play. I lost track of the instruments she brought to us, moving near to Catherine and I in turn, and playing over our prostrate forms. There was a rain stick which swirled and tumbled and made me think of shoals of fishes. There was singing, a Gayatri chant like those I'd heard sung at the mandir in Peterborough, something that I thought Christine called a 'happy drum' though I later discovered it was spelt 'HAPI', two sets of chimes, a djembe drum like those from Senegal that I'd learned to play, and a proper Rank Corporation-style gong that made me think of Mrs Dalloway's Big Ben and the 'leaden circles dissolving into air' with every stroke. Later Catherine described how she could visualise its sound moving around the room.

Apparently the variety of instruments is part of the approach to offering a sound bath – the lack of a fixed rhythm results in the brain not getting into a pattern, so that brainwave frequencies can be shifted. Each instrument was played for perhaps five minutes. After each there was a silence which I listened to, newly attuned. I heard Christine's Scholl sandals walking across the room to pick up the next instrument, the rasp of Velcro as she got a new instrument from its protective case.

I enjoyed lying down and listening to music and daydreaming (in the literature this is referred to as alpha brainwave state). I think I fell asleep – or what I'm told to refer to as theta wave state. But at only one point did the experience take me beyond what I feel I could have achieved lying on my bed listening to a world music CD of my choice – or any other beautiful sounds. Could there be similar benefit in a concert hall? In a church with its stentorian organ? (If so, perhaps the designers of the church had thought this through). Nevertheless, the moment which did distinguish the experience was like the opening of a door to a cinema showing a film I hadn't known was playing, startling in its clarity and powerfully elemental. But I could find no way to decode it. Even as someone who enjoys attempting to understand nighttime dreams as 'messages from our subconscious to our conscious minds' I was lost here. The image was only a fleeting moment but very vivid: a close-up of a breastfeeding child – mouth clamped round nipple. It was disconcerting and I was left wondering where on earth it came from and why. I didn't know whether in the image I was the baby or I was the breast – and if either of these, what the other was representing. I don't have, and haven't ever wanted, children, and have a straightforward relationship with my own mother. There was no narrative, no context, and once I'd been startled back to 'awake' there were no more striking images. I asked Christine about it and she said only that it was for me to understand.

Christine gave some feedback of her own experience of the session – that she had found lots of things we'd been 'holding' that we needed to get rid of. I thought of my rucksack which had been lugged on my journeys to get here like a reluctant travelling companion.

I asked whether Christine had done different things over me and over Catherine and she treated this like a silly question because 'of course' she did. Catherine apparently had more 'heavy' things so she had 'more gong work'. I was momentarily jealous.

Christine asked how we were feeling and Catherine talked about feelings of calm and peace, having been able to 'switch off' completely. She said that the sound baths always 'balanced' her, and having them on a Sunday night got her ready for the week, though at this point, right after the session, she felt 'spaced out and almost hypnotic, in a dreamlike state'. In a quick body-scan I couldn't honestly identify anything to report. Despite possibly having fallen asleep I felt neither refreshed nor drowsy. Christine, however, said that she could see us glowing. 'And I've cleaned up your little auras so they're all clear now,' she assured us like a cosmic charlady.

I wasn't sure whether I believed that I had an aura, but if I did I would really have liked it not to be a little one. However, a *clear* one had got to be a good thing, and as I shouldered on my rucksack at the end of the session I certainly felt lighter-headed. It's clever stuff.

I had a late bus back south and had to kill time in the city so I looked for a bar near the bus station and a way to say my farewells to Newcastle. Every bar I passed had disco ball lights (often more than customers now it was Sunday evening) or strobe effects, and wedding fave dance tracks. None of them were exactly what I wanted as a place to spend some quiet time on my own with a drink. I passed a subdued group of women who had perhaps come to the same conclusion. Maybe I could sit quietly in the lee of this group, who were huddled together and opening bottles of wine with what seemed more like duty or habit than enthusiasm. They had the weary team spirit of a group who had spent the weekend together.

'Well done, team,' said the woman managing the corkscrew. 'Nobody spewed.'

Gratitude diary entry
Rob's smile, and it being the first thing I saw on waking

Chapter 15

Iyengar Yoga – Maida Vale, London

'I think you could manage a shoulder stand'

If I'd walked out of Maida Vale station one afternoon in 1954 I might have passed two men chatting animatedly. One, at first glance a darker version of Charlton Heston, the other I might have recognised from posters as the celebrated violinist Yehudi Menuhin.

The station wouldn't have been much different from what I saw today – Maida Vale is one of London Underground's beautiful period-piece stations, clad in oxblood terracotta. An information board points out its vintage features, including the signage advertising a tobacconist's shop, noting that 'in fact the sign has outlived the shop itself!'.

It was just such a 'shop' that I was going to visit here – the Iyengar Institute where B K S Iyengar taught and which, even after his death, teaches the style of yoga which he developed, in the yoga tradition of knowledge passed down through a lineage from a guru. But this place is not only of relevance to followers of this school of yoga; thanks to those two ghosts I'd imagined hovering round the station it was the starting point for almost all approaches to postural yoga now popular in the UK – from chilly village halls to cool studios. This journey to the British mainstream started when Menuhin was in India in 1952, and Prime Minister Nehru introduced him to B K S Iyengar; the men's first meeting lasted three-and-a-half hours, while the friendship formed that day endured for decades. In 1954

Menuhin invited Iyengar to stay with him in Europe and teach him yoga – though the impact of his teachings was so holistic that at the end of that trip Menuhin gave him a watch engraved simply 'to my best violin teacher'. Menuhin became an advocate of yoga for all musicians, and yoga classes are still offered at the school he founded in Surrey.

However, even with Iyengar's visit to the UK, followers of his style of yoga here would have been limited to the musical elite if it had not been for a chance London dinner party conversation between Yehudi Menuhin's sister, Hephzibah, and Peter McIntosh, the then head of physical education in the Inner London Education Authority. McIntosh was interested in meeting the demand for yoga classes, but concerned not to have 'mystical' or 'spiritual' content paid for with government funds. Once McIntosh had investigated what Hephzibah had told him about Iyengar's methods he decided that this would be a suitable approach to offer for adult education courses. And so was born the 'yoga evening class', focusing on postures, and the direct line drawn from this London suburb to the Port Isaac village hall class and so many of the other experiences I'd had on this journey round British yoga.

Iyengar seemed an incongruous yoga guru from the images I'd seen of him – he had Ben Hur's strong face and barrel chest but carried on surprisingly skinny legs. I'd read that having been born during a flu pandemic, an attack left him sickly and later to struggle with malaria, tuberculosis and typhoid. He wrote in the *New York Times*:

> My arms were thin, my legs were spindly, and my stomach protruded… My head used to hang down and I had to lift it with great effort.

And yet this man had inspired not just a spiritual but an intense and precisely regulated physical discipline still followed today at his eponymous Institute and around the world.

My journey to the Institute led down a wide street lined with self-proclaimed 'mansions'. It reminded me of Alan Bennett talking of his childhood in Leeds where the same self-confident style of Edwardian domestic architecture had warped forever his vision of heaven as a place where his Sunday school teacher had told him 'my Father's house has many mansions'.

I didn't have long to walk through this heavenly vision before I came to an alley from which a young woman emerged in leggings and barefoot. There was no need for any other 'yoga happens here' sign.

Through a sheltered courtyard there was a small lobby for leaving your shoes, and an elegant reception area hung with photographs of BKSI and quotations from his works. I registered and paid my fourteen pounds and went into the beautiful teaching space. While nothing could rival the Brimham Rocks view, this was the most stunning setting I had yet practised in. It was the perfect physical representation of Iyengar's book's title; this was '*Light on Yoga*'. The room had twelve skylights and three clerestory windows. Glass bricks in the side walls and three long windows in the wall that the yoga mats faced towards contributed to the radiance that bathed the room. I thought of Iyengar's *Light on Life*:

> The hardness of a diamond is part of its usefulness, but its
> true value is in the light that shines through it.

With this stylish setting I could understand even better the following that Iyengar yoga has among the beautiful and lovers of beauty – famously including Annette Bening and Donna Karan. It gave an almost monastic atmosphere to the devotions within, but most of all it felt like an art gallery. I worried whether we were expected to be the works of art but took comfort from the spindly-legged wise man who knew about celebrating the channelling of light

For there was a theatrical rationale to this stark scene-setting; our eyes were guided to the light, and against the brightest wall was set a dais. It was to here that our teacher would come, and to this point that we would look for our enlightenment.

The tradition in which that teacher would work was made quite clear by the pictures hanging on the walls. There were eight pictures of BSKI, his hairless misproportioned body pliant in Triangle or Bridge. He had himself said of the building 'I feel I am part and parcel of this building from my heart, my head and my soul'.

To familiarise myself with what to expect here I had watched online an hour-long 1976 video of B K S Iyengar's practice. It had been billed as a yoga 'demonstration', and took place on a large and highly-patterned rug which gave it the air of being something filmed in someone's sitting room (I imagined it having been perhaps at the end of the sort of Maida Vale dinner party where Iyengar and the Menuhins might have been guests).

Iyengar had stood naked but for a pair of tartan briefs, over which discreet muffin tops bloomed. He gave an introduction on the freedom that comes with yoga, speaking in a doubly-distancing Indian version of a BBC accent.

I had been distanced, too, by his use throughout the recording of 'men'. The only time he mentioned women at all was when we were sat with legs splayed. 'This is a good pose for women too,' he noted, adding that with this pose pregnant women wouldn't have problems in labour. None of this appealed to my image of myself as a yogini.

It anyway wasn't the best thing to follow for home practice because of course it wasn't designed to be followed by anyone on the privacy of their laptop – it was recorded in the year the very first VHS machines were released – so there were no instructions given for anyone trying to copy the moves at home. I cricked my neck looking up to see what Iyengar was doing next. Most of the exercises were only done once – on the right or left – so I ended up feeling lopsided.

The 'demonstration' had started gently enough with standing in a star pose, moving into Triangle and a Warrior series. I followed gamely. There came a Sun Salutation – forward folds, back bends, Plank. I noted critically that Iyengar didn't even seem to be doing the poses particularly adeptly; to my surprise I felt I could have made suggestions for his alignment.

A Bind, Camel pose, Boat pose – this was all familiar and very doable for me. And then 'this is very good for sciatica', he had observed, and I listened up, having had twinges of this in recent months. Casually, Iyengar then put his leg around his neck, much as I might have adjusted my rucksack to sit more comfortably.

I had given up.

The rest of the session included a long time in headstand, along with Crane pose and many other ways that the *guruji*'s mastery became apparent. He was clearly a very strong man, even at the age of fifty-eight when the footage had been filmed.

Sitting on mats in the room here in Maida Vale, looking rather small in the face of such heritage, was the beginners' class of sixteen or so people, perhaps a quarter of them men, stretching and settling and massaging specific muscles like students about to sit an exam. Also dwarfing them was a terrifying looking wall garlanded with rope-like halters. I never found out what they were for, which only added to the fear they could inspire through the class.

While I was still stowing my bag, the door opened and the teacher came in. Seeing me standing up she asked, 'Who are you?'

I wasn't sure how to answer so I replied, 'I'm, er, Elizabeth.' She nodded, and I wasn't clear whether it had or had not been a satisfactory answer.

I hurried to take my place on my mat and the teacher looked out over the class. There were clearly other newcomers as she asked for more names. Her survey of the room reached the mat where I was now sitting in a half lotus and she asked again, 'What's your name?'

'I'm Elizabeth!' I said, rather more confidently this time and with a quizzical smile, which she did not return.

'Are you a beginner?' she asked.

'Not in yoga,' I said. 'But in Iyengar yoga, yes.'

She grimaced.

'Is that a bad thing?' I asked with a part-defiant, part-nervous laugh.

'Bad for you; not for me,' she said like a threat. She had an accent I couldn't place, so in fact she said it was 'bed for you' which sounded like I might end up hospitalised.

The repetition of my name in these two conversations didn't stop her from calling out to me later in the class when I needed to correct my positioning, 'hey, new girl in brown!'. It was a far cry from Ronna's personalised prayers for me or Karen's welcome in Cirencester.

The class started with three chanted *om*s, the room throbbing like a chapel with the shared reverberations. Then we were taken through some familiar poses but with each one broken down carefully into just what each part of our bodies should be doing in each. It felt like discipline, but – with the exception of when we were told to straighten our legs in a way that I'd always previously been told was hyperextension – it also felt good. The teacher placed great emphasis on stillness, so that once we were in a posture we just held it and breathed into it. In Downward-facing Dog, for example, there was none of the 'pedalling' of our feet that annoyed me.

'Be still!'

One of the men in the class had rippling upper body muscles. I sensed that our teacher saw him as a challenge. As we held a pose, he was rocking, each time pushing himself further into the position.

'This isn't the gym,' she told him, briefly.

She came off her dais – literally if not figuratively – and walked among us, stopping beside me to note that my feet were not parallel. Moving them as she instructed felt better. I wondered how many Dogs I'd held inaccurately without someone like her to guide me.

We moved through familiar poses of the Warrior sequence and Triangle pose, staring through those brilliant skylights and up at the heavens when our gaze followed our outstretched arms. Then we were each told to sit cross-legged facing the wall. It had overtones of the Naughty Step. With palms flat on it we pressed hard to develop muscle tone.

Next we were told to position ourselves a leg's length away from the wall, to turn our backs to it and bend from the waist, pushing our leg back so that a flexed foot made contact with the wall. Then we had to kick back against it.

She stopped at the fit young man a few mats down from me.

'You look like you're the age of my fourth child,' she said, 'and yet you can't do this...'

She beckoned to us all to gather round, and turned her toned and highly competent body into the position she'd been describing.

'Is there anyone here who's over eighty?' she asked. A polite laugh ran round the room.

'Then you can all do this.'

She gestured to the man who was the 'age of her fourth child' and the fair-haired girl next to me and told them to go back into the position. Obediently they did, though they were struggling. Despite the man's muscle (or perhaps because of it) he was stiff and inflexible.

'Look!' gestured the teacher at his unstraightened leg, and slapped it. 'Straighter, straighter!'

More laughter in the group but nervous now, feeling like we were colluding in something we didn't quite trust.

The fair-haired girl looked like she might be about to cry.

'It's embarrassing when young people can't even hold their leg straight,' the teacher said, and then sent us back to our mats. Since I was next to the girl I took the chance to mutter to her 'you did well' but she didn't acknowledge me. It wasn't my approval she wanted, and her rejection by our teacher had left her as shamed and inconsolable as a bullied child.

We went back into the next sequence and I was battling a juddering muscle when suddenly the teacher called out,

'Who tells you when to take a break?'

A girl at the front of the room had come out of the position and was sitting on her mat at rest.

'*I* tell you when to take a break,' she repeated, and the weary, embarrassed young woman obediently went back into position.

A *Yoga Journal* article about Iyengar gave some biography that helped to explain some of what might have been going on here. The sins of the father... the trauma of the guru... perhaps all these could be handed down generation to generation. And apparently when Iyengar was apprenticed to the yoga master Krishnamacharya, the apprenticeship was a tough one – once, when Krishnamacharya asked him to demonstrate Hanumanasana (a full split), Iyengar complained that he had never learned the pose. 'Do it!' Krishnamacharya commanded. Iyengar complied, tearing his hamstrings. I later watched an interview with Iyengar where he described his time with Krishnamacharya:

> He was creating fear complex in me more and more... that quality's in me because he did like that.

Iyengar went on to say that he himself nevertheless chose not to teach through fear, having experienced what it was like to have such a teacher, but I saw how seeds had been sown and perhaps were now flowering in this beautiful studio not just in the strengthening limbs and straining muscles of our group but in the quivering upper lip of my fellow yogini.

Next it was shoulder stand, which Iyengar called 'the mother of all the asanas', and the teacher walked around us dividing sheep from goats (these are not yoga poses). She came to me.

'I think you could manage a shoulder stand,' she said, and walked on.

I was ashamed at my jubilation, and knew it for the worst part of the experience under despotism. However much I had shrunk from the teacher's treatment of my classmates, however I had disagreed with her pedagogy – and her manners – she had established herself as top (upward-facing) dog and, like the pack animal I am, something deep within me had wanted her approval. And now she was saying she thought I could manage shoulder stand.

Which of course I knew. I'd done shoulder stand many times.

I tried to rationalise it to myself, that my reason for rejoicing was not her approval or permission, or the fact that I would do a shoulder stand – even though it is one of the positions I most enjoy in yoga; it was that I *looked* like someone who could do shoulder stand.

As usual, we worked into our shoulder stands by first going into Bridge, lying on the floor and lifting chest and hips until the former creates a chin lock. Holding myself here I knew I could easily get from here up into a shoulder stand. The teacher was passing by, and with my voice a little strangled by my own bosom I called to her tentatively.

'Can I go into shoulder stand?'

She acquiesced but even as I sent my toes up, stacking my vertebrae as I'd been taught, feeling – and beating – the tricks of gravity, I was furious with myself. As a full-grown adult I asked *permission* for my own body in my own time to move from one pose to another? It had taken me less than an hour to move from a functioning member of a democracy to an oppressed lackey of a totalitarian regime.

I'd been upside down for long enough; I started to feel the flickerings of blood's pressure around the edge of my eyeballs, and came back down. But I knew the cooling feeling of having been upside down, of having reversed my lymph flow, would continue to flow through me for the next thirty minutes.

After the shoulder stands it was time for headstands which I've never wanted to do, and probably don't have the strength to do properly. Headstands were one of Iyengar's signature poses. Famously, he taught them to Elisabeth, Queen of Belgium, when she was eighty, and after Iyengar's teaching, Yehudi Menuhin once conducted Beethoven's Fifth Symphony while standing on his head, directing the orchestra with his feet.

'New immigrants to that side,' said the teacher, so I and the other rawest of her recruits sat like the last to be picked for team sports, watching as the rest of the group took their positions as if in obeisance to the wall opposite us, and then flipped themselves up until their legs were against the wall. It was a strange display for us to be invited to watch, learning the tautness of buttocks, the way that breasts and bellies sag in unnatural directions with gravity pulling them from their proper place.

We didn't have long to muse on such inversions because soon we were back in a sequence for the whole class. The pace was slower now after the most energetic parts of the class had been completed. And the dictator on the dais was watching for our energy levels.

'You, blonde girl, need to rest,' she called out, and the wearied girl in question obediently went into Child's pose.

The only time I remembered seeing any like display of physical control and obedience was at a Bektashi Muslim celebration in Kosovo. The room there had been packed with devotees who stood (in Mountain pose, though they wouldn't have called it that) and rhythmically rocked back and forth, hitting themselves on the back with one hand as they did so. Over minutes and hours of this they worked themselves into a trance-like state and when one felt ready he would break free from his line and present himself on his knees before the 'Baba' leader of the community. If the Baba considered that a sufficient trance had been achieved he would then in a lightning move press a skewer clean through the supplicant's cheek. If his analysis had been correct then no blood flowed and the celebrant remained, pierced in a sign of his faith, amid the chanting and rocking robes of his congregation. In total perhaps a dozen men presented themselves in this way, all surveyed by the Baba who also identified when their trances might be wearing off, and when, with a swift brutal movement, he should withdraw the skewers and dismiss the man back to the lines of the other faithful. The lack of blood flowing down these mutilated cheeks was proof of the discipline and fanaticism. It had been the most terrifying and powerful religious experience of my life. Here in Maida Vale did not compare, but even the evocation was enough to make me work very hard at holding my poses.

I wanted to hate everything about my session. I wanted to hate the guru tradition that undermined my faith in myself and required me to put my faith in another, flawed person. I wanted to hate the powerplay that had led to people feeling inadequate. And yet...

Of all the classes I took, this was the one where the results lasted longest. I'm used to momentary euphoria after a yoga class, as endorphins and lactic acid rush in a heady cocktail through my body. I'm used to walking taller and more bouncily, and to feeling stretch – or ache – in my muscles the next day.

But after the Iyengar class the effects lasted for at least three days of feeling like I was living in a new body, an instrument of greater precision and greater power. In those days just doing ordinary things like taking steps along the street felt like exercises in poise and that there was the potential for more.

I made attempts at poses I had never tried before – in Plank I moved gecko-like by stretching out one arm to the side at a time; I even sank deep and trusting into the painful squat from which one launches into Crow, fixed my knees into my biceps and kicked slowly up with my feet, daring myself not to fall onto my skull. It was so obvious that falling onto my skull was what I was most likely to do, but I remembered Chris's reference to the 'conversation between your brain and your body' and tried not to place quite so much value on my precious, fragile, threatened brain. To my amazement and exhilaration, my body took over and I managed to hold myself like a louring dark bird in Crow pose for a few controlled, astounded seconds, before bringing my heels back down to earth.

I don't want to – really don't want to! – overclaim for Iyengar yoga or that particular class. My body had been undergoing lots of changes as I worked through this yoga journey. In the preceding six months I'd moved to an almost entirely vegan diet; I'd started paying attention to the medical recommendation of an hour's activity per day, and was getting up early to go for an hour's walk if I knew that the rest of the day would be sedentary; I had downloaded a program for my computer which made me stand up for at least a minute every hour; I'd started following a short YouTube video a few times a week with exercises for posture following seeing a shocker of a photograph of myself stoop-shouldered... I was overhauling my funny old body in lots of new ways at once. But it did feel that the day I did Iyengar yoga was the day that marked a step change; towards something like what Iyengar himself had described in his *Light on Life* book – that 'it is through your body that you realise you are a spark of divinity'.

'You look ... strong,' said a friend I'd not seen in a couple of years as soon as I walked into the café to meet her.

'Yogic-bodied' was the word used by another friend who'd seen me a few months before and who knew about my project.

I felt supple and healthy. I had lost weight: I could feel my sitting bones when I was seated. I discovered new contouring on my thighs, with definition in places I'd thought would always be rag-doll-rounded. I felt like I had taken off a thick and not very well-designed trouser suit. I felt freer, with a new sense of this body I lived with, lived in, lived through. I had a new feeling of my body as a creation of muscle and bone – yes, with some fat plumping it out in places, but that as incidental. I've been thinner – I had jackets and trousers which reminded me of that when I confidently stepped into them – but I didn't think I'd ever been fitter.

Gratitude diary entry
my new bamboo socks that are soft and sustainable

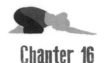

Chapter 16

Yoga Nidra – Stroud

'Listen to your body like you would to an old friend'

I walked up a lane to a garden where about fifteen young women were sitting on a sun-dappled lawn in poses suggesting various stages of enlightenment.

I had come to this house on the outskirts of Stroud for a whole day's experience, which would include my first taste of yoga *nidra*. 'One hour of yoga nidra is worth four hours of normal sleep' the internet had explained to me, and the course – with these miraculously restorative exercises – was to be led by the co-founder of the Yoga Nidra Network. The idea of a whole day of yoga appealed more than the hit-and-run of yoga quickies in studios where you didn't have to do anything other than yoga. Here we would also eat lunch (mindfully) and talk to one another (yogically), and I felt that I might come to some more profound learning as a result.

But unlike the classes I'd done where you could shuffle in and sit on your mat in silence, I sensed that today was therefore going to require some interaction from me.

'Should I sit here?' I asked the women on the grass and those who didn't have their eyes fixed on some far-off inner or outer drishti nodded vaguely at me.

I felt square. I had used the word 'should'. But I did want to know whether I was kind of in the right place. *Ahh, but wherever you are is the 'right' place* said an irritating dopey voice inside me.

And there wasn't just me; there was my enormous rucksack to consider. I was not travelling light; that, too, made me feel square. I said no more, but took the rucksack off and sat down on the grass. I kept a nice straight back but I didn't form a mudra with my hands.

There was silence.

Looking around me I decided I had better take off my shoes too. I sat back down.

I wondered who these people were. Had they been here before? Had they stayed here last night? I knew it would help me settle if I could know something about them, and I also knew that you have a tiny window if you really want to be the one who talks in a silent group: silence like a cancer grows.

'So,' I cleared my throat and attempted unoriginally, 'have you all been here before?'

Before anyone could answer, an energetic woman hurried out of the house with a tray of mugs. I relaxed. Now the person who was in charge was here and I would find out what to do.

You don't have to do *anything; you don't have to* be *anyone* said the joss-stick-husky voice in my head.

Uma was talking over the voice as she set down the tray.

'If you want the toilet, I do really urge you to use the back garden,' she said. 'I honestly think that our golden stream is one of the offerings we can make to Mother Earth and a connection we can make with her. So feel free to go round the back. You can dry your yoni in the wind.

'Of course, if you actually like pissing in drinking water then you can use the indoor bathroom, but I invite you to think about that.'

I wasn't going in that back garden, I was sure about that.

But did I want to be marked out as a pisser in drinking water? I didn't think I was going to use the indoor bathroom either.

It seemed like I wouldn't be *going* anywhere today.

With sanitary instructions issued, Uma left the teapot and the tray of mugs and hurried off.

I resisted the urge to organise the tea-drinking, and another woman started passing the mugs round and pouring us each a curl of witchy cinnamony steam. I lowered my face to it and inhaled.

It was true, I did not have to do anything or be anyone. I sat and drank the tea in silence.

Soon we were invited inside the yoga space – an outbuilding just across the garden. Inside, we found the walls lined with shelves holding books whose spines were colour-coordinated. I was by the blue-indigo-violet section with books on Picasso, Iyengar, *The Sutras of Patanjali, What to Expect When You're Expecting*, Shere Hite: Uma is also known as the developer of 'womb yoga'.

I thought of the monkish emptiness of the Iyengar Institute. Yoga was certainly a broad church, with beautiful empty chapels and other, more cluttered, locations where you were invited to piss on the lawn.

To prepare for the nidra we each found a yoga mat to settle onto, and began snuggling in among the sheepskin rugs and pashminas and Indian silk bolsters we had all been given. A woman who was heavily pregnant was struggling to get comfortable and Uma went over to her and propped and manipulated her like a midwife might. 'How's that?'

'It's OK,' came a muffled voice from someone who sounded like she had resigned herself nearly nine months ago to the fact that she might never be comfortable again.

'We can do better than OK,' insisted Uma, shifting her and positioning bolsters more carefully. The pregnant yogini sighed deeply.

'Ohh, that's really good.'

Once all fifteen of us were settled in our little burrows, we waited for the show to start. I felt as ignorant and tense as a Victorian girl on her wedding night. My eyes roved around the room, looking for clues as to what might be about to happen here.

In between the shelves were geometric shapes painted onto the plaster. I had recently learned that these were called *yantras*, mystical diagrams from the Tantric traditions used for the worship of deities or as an aid in meditation (and yes, some of them do have words written on them to be repeated, making them Tantra mantra yantras. These were the thoughts I was occupying myself with before our nidra began).

'Nidra' is the Sanskrit word for 'sleep' and we were basically being invited to a long, deep nap. It had been many decades since I'd last lain in a room with others and been requested to go to sleep, but in this callback to nursery school Uma started us with some standard relaxation – focus on our breathing, and a body scan. As usual we were invited to clear our minds, but Uma's approach struck me. First of all she said,

'We don't need to be mind masters.'

I felt muscles perceptibly slacken. Oh, phew. We didn't!

'The mind will go on thinking, because that is what she does,' said Uma.

The impact of that pronoun was striking. I thought of that Peterborough monk nine hundred years ago dipping pen in ink and writing her down. It did make a difference; language did matter.

Uma's nidra was in a mixture of a language which may have been Hindi or Sanskrit or any other language I don't know, combined with English with surprise Estuary accents and glottal stops. It was all blended with music from a squeezebox and a gong, and singing in half-notes from Uma's colleague Sivani. In between the singing, Uma muttered rhythmically, extemporising like a playful yoga rapper, the repeated mantra was 'I honour my heart, my inner teacher'.

'Listen to your body,' said Uma, 'like it's your best friend.'

It was a startling idea. I did listen to my body, but much of the time I did so as if it was an annoying, if sometimes loveable, toddler:

'Oh please stop whining; if we can keep going for a little bit longer I'll buy you an ice cream.'

'Time for beddy-bies is it?'

But like my best friend? What would it say to me if I listened like that; *I'm really hungry*, I heard my body say. I knew my new veganism was taking a toll. And then, quieter, almost pleading, *Oh, Elizabeth. I'm also just really, really... tired.*

I discovered tears running down my face.

I regained a hold of myself when we did some focused breathing, and as Uma led us in a deep breath out, our exhalation was joined by the sound of a train hurtling along the nearby line to Cheltenham, its whistle streaming. Perhaps, like Allan Quatermain in *King Solomon's Mines* tapping into his knowledge of the eclipse, Uma scheduled her teaching in this space to coordinate with the train timetable.

At the end we were gently brought back to reality by Uma walking round the room and fanning us. I opened my eyes and saw the flapping wing of a big black bird above me. No apparition, this was a genuine raven's wing she was using. This felt like a dark place to succumb to sleep.

I don't know how long the nidra lasted – maybe no more than twenty minutes; maybe an hour. At the end I felt relaxed, but sluggish rather than re-energised. But the other women in the room were making yummy noises like people who'd just had an excellent meal or some deeply nurturing experience; a long cuddle perhaps.

Gently we were invited to sit back up. Uma invited us each to say a bit about ourselves; why we were here, what had come up for us in the nidra. I wasn't the only person to have been brought to tears by being here. A box of tissues that I noticed was labeled 'man-size' was passed round as the group shared the diverse journeys and dreams that had brought them to this space and this day. Women had come from all over the country and even beyond; here were the types I had got used to spotting – I made silent namaste to the tattooed girl with blue hair and to another recurring yogini, with unshaved legs and painted toes. I could understand and celebrate either one of these as a style or lifestyle choice, but the combination seemed contradictory.

After each contribution everyone made a little namaste sign with their hands in gratitude. I remembered how hard I'd found it to say 'namaste' at all when I started yoga, wondered how I still found it necessary to use an exclamation mark after it when I signed an email to anyone in the yoga world, and how I heard the inverted commas in my head on the rare occasions I spoke the word. I had moved from feeling it as an affectation, to genuine love and learning for what it meant in recognising both the 'divine light' (yes, I still needed the inverted commas round words like *divine*) in me and that in the other person – whatever challenges they were currently presenting me with.

But now I was as self-conscious as I'd been in that first yoga class, and I could not form my hands into prayer position fifteen times. I smiled instead.

Uma said she would now lead us through some physical asanas and I imagined listening to my 'old friend' on this. Yes, she was up for some movement after the grogginess of our post-nidra state and the cloying smell of geranium oil which Uma had passed round until we were all scented like Turkish delight. So we stood up and had the chance to stretch in some gentle asanas, I tried moving through them while listening all the time to my 'friend'.

Oh, that feels good.

I'm going to go deeper into this pose.

Ouch! Don't push me like that.

And then came one which I knew my friend wouldn't like.

'Plant your feet on the ground,' Uma instructed. 'And now lift the three middle toes up.'

I couldn't do this. There's something in the wiring of my body; some fine motor control that might have blighted my life if it had been in the muscles of mouth or hand, but in my case is in the toes. I stood back while everyone else wriggled their metatarsals expertly. Uma saw me withdraw.

'Oh, I just can't do this,' I explained.

'Yes, you can if you try,' she said with the same persistence that had eventually had her settling the pregnant woman so comfortably before the nidra.

'No, it's just something in my wiring,' I said with the confident expertise of the person who had been guiding this particular machine for over forty years.

'Try holding down the big toe and the little toe with your hand,' she said with the confident expertise of someone who had been watching people wiggle their appendages in this yoga space for decades.

I followed what she said, forcing my uncooperative toes like restraining a large hallucinating patient, and watched my middle toes eventually and rather miraculously respond.

'Now take your hand away, and now the toes know what they're doing, lift up those middle ones on their own.'

It's not often at the age of forty-four that you watch your body learn a new skill – especially one that is usually learned in childhood. Admittedly my toes didn't lift very far, and the left foot struggled much more than the right, but I could see neurological rewiring taking place before my eyes.

Then I took my 'friend' to lunch (she asked for seconds of the fragrant curry). I talked to the other participants about nidra practice, and a woman called Yasmine told me she did a nidra twice a day as the only way she could manage her fibromyalgia and ME. Her fourteen-year-old son does it too. Another woman said her children do it on a daily basis too, and that she always does it before bed.

Over the food, helping each other to more vegetables, we gently shared our stories – our frailties, the things we wanted to learn, the people we wanted to love, the roads we were travelling. I had been right about the qualitative difference in the experience of a day-long course; perhaps I hadn't felt the restorative powers of the nidra but sitting comfortably among these women dressed in a rainbow of earth colours I thought of Chaucer's pilgrims and felt lucky with what I had gained. If I was on a yoga journey, then the other yoga experiences had been petrol-station-stop opportunities to refresh and refuel. Today, while I was still certainly in transit, I felt I had joined a caravan. And, most importantly, here I had found a new travelling companion to listen to on my onward travels – I had reunited with an old friend.

Gratitude diary entry
the privilege of waking in the art studio of a friend where a bed had been put up for me, surrounded by the evidence of her creativity

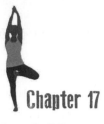

Chapter 17

Children's Yoga – Slough

'There can be a lot of people who are very stressed in school
and they get annoyed with things'

Yasmine, whom I'd met in Stroud, had told me she had been
doing yoga since she was a thirteen-year-old in care. What she'd
learned there had seen her through the horrors of her adolescence –
with an absent father and a bipolar mother – as well as through ME
as an adult.

I'd assumed she'd started her practice as part of a project for
youngsters like her but no, she said, she'd had to find the class herself.
When a kid has been left without functional parents, I thought that
the least we could do would be to offer them the tools to patch together
self-care and self-confidence. I hoped that the next generation of
youngsters would be better off than Yasmine and looked for a chance
to see children's yoga in practice in this country. The best place to do
so would surely be the youngest city in Britain; so where do you think
that is?

The answer may surprise you. It certainly surprised the people I
spoke to when I went there. But according to the Centre for Cities,
the UK's youngest city is Slough, with an average age of 33.9 and only
one in ten people aged 65 or over.

Arriving in Slough by train, the first thing you see is evidence of
the babies it feeds. The Horlicks factory with its Art Deco clock and
monotype signage is a landmark for anyone travelling on that stretch of

track into or out of London's Paddington station. I'd admired the site, drunk the drink, and even modified the drink (my turmeric Horlicks might not yet be market-ready but my maltshakes are crowd-pleasers), but until coming to Slough I hadn't known that Horlicks had started life as a baby food – patented in 1873, and only later sold for adults 'to give the fitness and stamina that prevents undue fatigue'.

The retro factory was the last stylish thing I saw for a while, however, as I wandered through a deserted shopping mall. Outside Superdrug a young guy was using his smartphone to take a picture of an advertised sales assistant vacancy. I couldn't decide if it was an image of aspiration or of desperation.

I'd read that Slough's unemployment rates were a third of the national average, and that it had the highest number of global corporate headquarters outside of London; this place should feel booming, but I wandered past Moneygram offices, pawnbrokers, pound shops and their nutritional equivalent in fast food outlets – including the intriguing Mr Chicken Bites (noun or verb?).

I was going to visit a class of yoga for children run by Kalyani. She'd told me that she started as a yoga teacher for adults, but had then seen what it could offer her own three children and the children of the parents who attended her classes, so earlier this year she started a class for kids. She described the classes as offering children 'a new confidence in their bodies, and yoga techniques that will act as a friend to them for the rest of their lives'.

Her sessions take place out of town so I got a taxi which took me to the Community Centre where the class was to be held with plenty of time to spare. While waiting I tried to learn something about Berkshire's children and the community into which they were born. The noticeboards were an index of rich opportunities: belly dancing;

Pilates; a Pop Quiz and Party in aid of the mental health charity, Mind; baby sign language; Brahma Kumaris, which I intended to find out more about; Weight Watchers; and ballet. There were photographs on display of the two-way street at the Centre of any Community — as well as the opportunities you *get* there was evidence of the opportunities people *gave* to others, with pictures showing adult and child volunteers painting the corridors.

The noticeboards presented an image of an ideal community, and as if to prove it, I read that *Midsomer Murders* had been filmed at the nearby airfield. British television rarely puts a greater seal of approval on a rural community than staging a fictional murder there.

And these noticeboards were a beautiful illustration, too, of just what could be meant by the public information poster also on display, outlining Slough's initiative to stop people being drawn into radicalisation (only the previous year a local man had been jailed for spreading ISIS propaganda). The poster trumpeted the importance of understanding that 'your opinions count', of individual liberty, and of tolerance.

The leaflets available also gave information about the nearby White Waltham parish which prided itself not on youth but on age — a yew tree in the churchyard reputed to be over a thousand years old. Its Great Wood is 'home to a variety of birdlife, and the migrating hobby is known to nest there'.

Indeed the migrating hobby was really something of a tradition in Slough — from the Welsh who arrived in the 1930s to the Polish who settled from nearby refugee camps after the Second World War, and more recent arrivals. It is now one of the most ethnically diverse towns in Britain, with a population that is forty-six per cent White, forty per cent Asian, and nine per cent Black.

But above all, the centre showed the practical implications of Slough's young population and the range of needs that such a population might have. Special activities for 'twins and multiples'; advice for parenting during and after domestic violence; a nurture group offering jelly play, water play and an appetising-sounding 'peas and sweetcorn' session; and a Maternity Network leaflet listing people around Slough who could help with pregnancy reflexology, baby portraits, baby and toddler swimming lessons, postnatal personal training, doulas and lactation consultancy, among other things. Kids needed a lot of help to get into the world, and stay healthy once they got there. And I knew they needed yoga.

In the local Family Information and Leisure Guide, available free of charge, I wondered whether yoga opportunities might be listed. I looked up ideas for 'Rainy days and when funds for outings are low'. Yoga was not mentioned, as these seemed to be rainy days from the last century, and the best advice in that section was to 'use doilies for pretty paintings'. I think there's now an app for that.

And with this I had pretty much exhausted the public information literature available for Slough's families and was ready to meet them in person. I was grateful when children started to arrive for Kalyani's session.

In the end there were nine children (all but one were girls) plus one mum taking part in the class. All seemed calm and confident in their practice. Four were of Indian heritage and their ages ranged from five to fourteen; Kalyani said she thought society was 'too split up' and that having a full age mix was a benefit.

As they took their places on their mats, some slipped naturally into Child's pose – the position where it had taken me six years of yoga to be able to get heels and buttocks to touch. One of the children settled happily in the pose before me now had only six years of existence; it was a vivid reminder that sometimes you're better at things before you start practising them.

The class opened with a mantra in Sanskrit. Kalyani gave me a card with its translation:

> *Om*, may God protect us together. May he accept and
> nourish us together. May we work together with great vigour.
> Let our learning shine brightly. Let there be no discord
> amongst us. *Om*. Peace, peace, peace.

It was pretty full on for a six-year-old, but the children chanted gamely along. The mother who was accompanying her daughter sat behind her with hands in prayer pose and they chanted *om* precise octaves apart. Later she told me about the connection yoga was making for her and her daughter.

Afterwards Kalyani confirmed that her teaching for children is no different from what she teaches adults. I asked whether any of the parents had queried the religious aspect around the edges of the yoga taught here. I'd read a recent Office of National Statistics report which showed that religious devotion in Slough was the highest in the country, and I was pretty sure that most of the children in the group weren't from a Hindu background. Kalyani said she'd had no comments. 'I just want people to know there is something bigger than us, to connect with the light within us and with others. Personally, yoga has helped me connect with my Hindu faith.'

The class was underway when two latecomers arrived. They were Year Seven girls and they walked in with attitude. I thought of Yasmine from Stroud and was so glad these 'whatever' girls were here.

Kalyani talked the children through focusing on their breath. The power of this is a simple, even boring, message to share; it doesn't bring the rush of blood to the head that you get in a shoulder stand or Plough; the Instagram Insta-gratification of Tree or Dancer, the playfulness of Happy Baby or Lion, the pride and awe at your body's endless possibilities that you get from Crow. How would this go down with a group of children? I looked at their faces, earnestly tracing the movement of breath through their body, some with a small frown like I'd seen kids use at their Xbox on working through a particularly tricky level. There was of course one girl who was still knotting her T-shirt – and she was probably the one who needed the breath awareness most.

Kalyani spiced it up a bit by suggesting that they imagine the breath coming in coloured a gleaming gold; these kids were being given an extraordinary gift. As Ajay, the twelve-year-old boy currently observing the rise and fall of his chest, told me later, 'Like it's before something important and you can't sleep then breathing helps, and focusing on different parts of your body.' Thirteen-year-old Charlotte said this was the thing she most values from the class – 'The deep breathing helps. Let's say I'm in a situation like homework then I can take a deep breath.' I thought again of Yasmine and the strength she'd found in a damaged childhood, and I wished it to all these fragile children.

Kalyani mentioned the twelve Thai boys who'd been in the news a few weeks before when they were trapped in an underground cave with their football coach for more than two weeks before their miraculous rescue. The boys, aged eleven to seventeen, had apparently used meditation to help them. The thought of trying to focus like this in the craggy grip of a dripping cave forced a stoniness around my tender claustrophobic heart. Looking at these kids, the same age as the stranded Thai footballers, I felt again the vulnerability of childhood, the need to offer them all not just wetsuits and face masks, but more enduring rescue gear.

Kalyani moved the group into the day's asanas, with stretches on either side. The T-shirt-knotter had difficulty following these, too, so she was on the wrong side each time. It meant that as the children stretched their legs out to the side she could tickle the toes of her neighbour with her own. She did so.

Then Kalyani gave the children a challenge – to get from sitting to standing without using your hands. In fact that was the first yoga for children I had ever come across – on my teaching practice in a London school I helped in a class run by a supply teacher of Indian origin. Supply teachers have a literal and metaphorical bag of tricks to keep the attention of children enjoying the opportunities of someone being in charge of their class who doesn't know the rules, hardly knows their names, and is usually too scared to ask for help. This supply teacher had clearly had a yoga favourite, and I saw with admiration how it engaged the bodies and brains of a group of ten-year-olds in the dangerous 2.30pm lull. The kids in Kalyani's class were just as engaged.

Sitting on the floor of the sports hall, I had a go myself. I felt the tightening of my core, the lift in my thighs. I bruised my knees... I was no good at this. Indeed I've been practising ever since. It seemed like an easy way to incorporate some muscle tone into the sedentary bits of my lifestyle so now I take up Kalyani's challenge every time I stand up. And I've since read research (in the *European Journal of Preventive Cardiology*) that being able to do this is a good predictor of life expectancy. In their study of men and women aged fifty-one to eighty, those who needed to use both hands and knees to get up and down (whether they were middle-aged or elderly) were almost seven times more likely to die within six years. So bruise away, knees!

The children were told to get 'onto all fours' to move into the spine-bending Cat and Cow postures.

T-shirt-mangler thought about this.

'Why is it called *all fours*?' she asked. It was a good question, which I'd never thought about before. You could call Downward-facing Dog 'all fours' since there were four points of contact with the ground. Or Bridge pose, for that matter, where you again have four points of contact with the ground, though it's your back rather than your front which is facing the floor. And with the word 'all' it suggested that you'd be lying the length of your limbs down. And while we're on the subject, why the plural? Why not 'get down on *all four*'?

Nobody answered her and eventually she got on with arching her back with the rest of them.

From here they moved into Warrior I, arms raised above their head with legs in a lunge. 'Feel strong in your warrior,' said Kalyani.

They moved back into Mountain pose and then they were told to prepare to jump into Warrior II. I've moved into Warrior II on a regular basis for the last eleven years and never felt much excitement about it, but now a ripple of anticipation ran through the class. Together they jumped and shouted 'WARRIOR!'. It definitely made it more fun that way.

The Year Seven girls were fully taking part now, and afterwards when I spoke to one of them she mentioned this move as a highlight – 'You go 3-2-1 then "boom" and I feel like everything's coming out – the stress and anger of homework or exams.'

Then they moved to the wall where they did star poses – right foot and right arm on the ground while their left arms and legs were in the air.

'Ow,' said one of the girls.

'We don't like *ows* in yoga,' Kalyani reminds her.

From here it was an easy move to Downward-facing Dog against the wall and into a handstand.

One of the Year Seven girls was struggling.

'I can't,' she said.

Kalyani was calm again. 'Have a bit more faith in yourself. Do it slowly and tell yourself you can do it.'

When I looked up again, the girl was upside down, and smiling.

The session was coming to an end and Kalyani asked whether the children had any requests. The popular choices were a surprise – Pigeon (ouch!), Crow (ouch, ouch!), Bird of Paradise (standing with one leg in the air, cradled by arms, one behind it and one in front; ooh!), Plough and Sphinx.

'We can't do them all,' said Kalyani. 'We have to finish soon; we've got karate coming.'

Such are the realities of practice in a community centre.

After the class I had the chance to talk to some of the children. The most inspiring were that Year Seven pair of self-identified 'besties'.

'Some friends think it's cool; some think it's weird,' they said, which fits with my own experience of people's perceptions of yoga. But they talked confidently about how it helped them relax and how 'it was easy to join because people are welcoming'. But more importantly, they talked about the attitudes it had changed in them – it was the main thing they do out of school but 'you might as well give things a go – like that handstand'. I remembered Kalyani's voice, 'Have a bit more faith in yourself. Do it slowly and tell yourself you can do it'. It's a voice most of us could have done with hearing when we were on the brink of puberty.

As Ajay added, 'It would be a good thing to start in schools. There can be a lot of people who are very stressed in school and they get annoyed with things.'

There can be, and they can do. And yoga can't cure it all – it couldn't bring back Yasmine's father or make the youngsters' exams go away. But listening to these wonderfully earnest children – the T-shirt knotter, the *besties* and all – talking about what their yoga meant to them it seemed they had a better chance of triumphing than the rest of those tens of thousands now growing up in this young town.

Gratitude diary entry
waking to an email from a friend asking to meet up

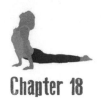

Chapter 18

Brahma Kumaris – on the Isle of Man

'If you're feeling seasick, go down into the engine room'

I was nervous about getting seasick. I had arrived for my short stay on the Isle of Man by aeroplane but the prices were prohibitive for flights back to the mainland – or 'across' as I would learn to call it here, in terminology which seemed vaguely euphemistic. You might as well call it 'passing over'. So to go 'across' and back to England I would have to take a ferry. Based on my previous seafaring experiences it might turn out to be very like dying.

I shared some of these thoughts with the taxi driver who picked me up from the airport. He was cheerful, but not just blithely optimistic (as it emerged he had been when he estimated what the taximeter would run to). His positivity about my return crossing – may I rest in peace – turned out to be informed by him having previously worked as an engineer on the Isle of Man Steam Packet Company. I learned that after nearly 190 years, the company is the oldest continuously operating passenger shipping company in the world. But yes, the boats were modern enough. Nevertheless, he admitted that things could get 'lumpy'.

'But if you're feeling seasick, go down into the engine room.'

I laughed politely, with a stomach already churning at the idea of adding in diesel fumes to my queasiness.

'No, I'm serious. It might sound mad, but when I was an engineer on the boats, no matter how bad things were up above, I would go down into the engine room and I would hardly notice we were moving. It was only when my spanner fell out of my hand and bounced around that I knew we had a rough crossing.'

I listened carefully as I had come to the Isle of Man to try Raja yoga, a way to achieve 'meditative consciousness' or access to my own engine room, even when the tides around were turbulent. This is not a 'Hatha', or asana-focused, approach to yoga so there would be no physical poses or exercises; instead there was a focus on the 'limbs of yoga' related to focused concentration, meditative absorption, and perhaps even *samadhi* – enlightenment. However, the Pradipika says 'Raja yoga will not be complete without Hatha, nor Hatha without Raja yoga', so what I learned here should contribute to, and be influenced by, everything else I was learning in the physical parts of my yoga journey.

The Raja yoga courses are run as part of the Brahma Kumaris worldwide spiritual movement 'dedicated to personal transformation and world renewal'. There are Brahma Kumaris centres in 110 countries, and activities at over 40 locations in the UK, so the choice of the Isle of Man was not forced on me. Islands have a distinct spiritual pull, however, and the idea of one poised almost equidistant between England, Ireland and Scotland, an island whose very name suggested it could tell us something about our fundamental nature, had attracted me. It seemed this was a place of contemplation: the island's tourist information promotes the opportunities for stargazing that result from its low light pollution; it has the largest cluster of 'dark sky discovery sites' in the British Isles.

But alongside this instinct about the island as a place to meditate, I had very little information about it – not much more than its flag (with one leg too many) and its most famous mammal (with one tail too few). The taxi ride from the airport filled me in on more. The driver's headlines were the drugs problem ('nothing else to do') and the lack of a speed limit on the unrestricted roads.

It seemed like a dangerous mix, but he went on to describe – with the passion that maybe only a professional driver could have – what the derestriction meant on these winding roads.

'I know that's not unique: the German autobahns are unrestricted too, but what you're driving on there is cut *through* the land; here the roads work *with* the land.' It was a strangely hippy approach to fast cars.

And of course the speed along the island's roads was another thing I did know about the Isle of Man: though I'd never actually watched the TT ('tourist trophy') motorcycle races, it's the only activity I knew of taking place on the island. Over the next few days I saw signs of it everywhere – in the temporary seating built into embankments on particularly exciting turns and in motorcycling memorabilia in shops catering for tourists. With 45,000 visitors each year arriving on the island just for the race, it accounts for one sixth of tourist numbers. Joanna, who would be running the meditation class, had told me that they'd not been able to hold the meditation session the previous week 'because it was TT week'. It was a part of the calendar of island life, like Christmas or the harvest.

As our driver talked I was listening out for an Isle of Man accent, trying to imagine what a blend of Scots, Irish and Scouse might sound like. It seemed a lot like Yorkshire to me.

'Yeah, my mum brought me and my brother here from Sheffield when I was seven!'

As I continued my careful listening out for an accent over the days on the island I was thwarted every time. I heard Estuary English, Glaswegian, Filipino and more. Eventually I realised that these might in fact be the most 'typical' Manx accents – in the latest census the percentage of those born 'on-island' was (by a tailless cat's whisker) for the first time less than the percentage of the so-called 'comeovers' (49.8:50.2 per cent). The member of the Brahma Kumaris community I spoke to who had come here from Zimbabwe told me about the 10,000 South Africans on the island – an extraordinary population in an island of only 83,000 people.

I was starting to see the island not as the place of retreat I had imagined but as a place of union and connections with a wider world. The next day I was told about a pineapple-canning factory in the Philippines which had recently mechanised. Laid-off staff were apparently being brought over to prop up the Manx health service, which was reeling from new regulations that made it hard for NHS staff to transfer their pension, and thus a shortage of British medical staff willing to work on the island. It's a rather wonderful world when a pineapple tin seals on one hemisphere and a door opens for a Filipino care worker on a wind-blown island on the other. And it seems that the island has always been well-connected – when we visited the cathedral in Peel I learned that even back in the Middle Ages, when you might have thought that globalisation had not yet been invented, the island had been part of the diocese of Trondheim, thirteen hundred kilometres away in Norway. Later I heard about the tailless Manx cat population that had even reached Denmark, brought there by ship. Perhaps mainlanders always overestimate the isolation of an isle.

Of course the mainlanders like me were the other factor that joined up the island. But the numbers of us coming over as tourists are in something of a crisis now – approximately half what they were in the late 1940s when half a million people would come over each year to engulf the small island population. At the time of my journey there were newspaper headlines about a slump in the latest visitor numbers that were the worst for a decade.

Though that's exactly what attracts some people – a 1904 official guide I'd found suggested the town where we'd be staying, Peel, as 'an ideal resting-place for the toil-worn worker from the hurrying outer world'. And there were signs everywhere of the island's Otherness and seclusion from the hurrying outer world. Here we were in the British Isles, but not in Great Britain, or even the United Kingdom. As a British Crown Dependency, cars do not have British number plates, websites have their own domain ending; my UK mobile didn't work here without going into roaming, and local people explained that they have to buy health insurance to cover them if they want to go 'over' to the Kingdom, where a Manx passport won't get you NHS coverage; the coins were different (I got used to receiving change in loaghtan sheep, shearwaters and cats, and though mainland currency was accepted here, the Manx round pounds were useless to me on my return at the end of my visit) and when I went to buy a second-class stamp at the independent Isle of Man Post Office I was told with dignity 'our mail is all first class. *And* it only costs 52p'.

I was looking forward to exploiting the island's opportunities to leave some old habits behind, en route to a New World. But before I went to the Brahma Kumaris centre I was to spend a few nights in what was technically the Isle of Man's only city, Peel (population: 5,000). Searching Peel's online tourist guidance before my visit I had picked up an air of melancholy in a place with the soubriquet 'sunset city', like a retirement home, and which was referred to on one bravely enthusiastic website as having been 'once practically the kipper-smoking capital of the world'.

It is a sleepy city. It was here that I learned my only Manx phrase, '*traa dy liooar*' meaning 'time enough'. I found it written on brass plates screwed to the benches along the cliff path into town when I went walking the next morning, and it seemed everywhere, infusing the unhurried approach to the service of my salad of local crab (though perhaps the poor crab might not have agreed with it), and the casual chattiness of staff and customers in every shop.

The chattiness helped for getting a handle on the island's history. I started at the bookshop ('A Novel Experience'). This was sleepy to the point of risking bankruptcy and as I leafed through the Local Interest section I asked the friendly owner for some more information about this place. We seemed to have *traa dy liooar*, but I couldn't even pronounce it, so I opened with some questions about the language. Was it dying?

'Oh no,' he assured me. Although there hadn't been a native speaker of Manx alive since the 1970s, recently a primary school had opened offering education all in the Manx language. 'Yeah, so my friend now has three teenage daughters who share a secret code… Can you imagine? My friend is having to learn the language now,' he grinned.

He told me about working for the local library service part-time, and it was on my stop at the city library later that I found a Reader's Digest guide to *The World's Religions; Understanding the Living Faiths* and, under 'Hinduism and Sikhism', some sketchy details of the Brahma Kumaris movement. It said it was 'founded in 1937 in Hyderabad by a diamond merchant' – the diamonds seem to be mentioned in most descriptions of the BK. Sometimes the reference is admiring ('imagine! He had all that and chose to focus on meditation'); sometimes it seems to invite skepticism ('how unworldly can such a man really be?'). But

about the diamond geezer himself I could find out very litt
the next day's session still felt like a mystery.

In the meantime I covered some more familiar religious ground, with a visit to Peel Cathedral. I discovered it in the middle of a huge new garden planting project with banners explaining how the investment aimed to meet 'the needs of faith tourism' on the island. As well as the cathedral's Viking links they referenced the Catholic heritage of Rushen Abbey in Ballasalla and the Celtic heritage of Maughold. Perhaps unsurprisingly, they didn't mention my own personal site of pilgrimage to the Brahma Kumaris centre, but I suddenly started feeling like I was part of a tradition. Get me, a faith tourist!

But still a tourist because the day's greatest excitement came with the cat. It was sitting on a step with all evidence of its taillessness – or not – hidden under it. I stood watching, willing it to get up so I could discover whether it was a 'rumpy', 'stumpy' or 'longy' in the self-explanatory taxonomy of Manx cats. Eventually – and with disdain – it raised itself up in a beautiful vinyasa, and swayed past me waving its behind to reveal that there was... nothing there!

The next day was when I had to make the bus trip to Douglas so I could be there for the Raja yoga class in the evening. It was the kind of day when you need meditation – I'd woken up to a string of challenging emails, including one from a colleague with a description of a mistake I'd made with gentle, fair and precise details (they're the worst) and another from someone who'd got hold of my password (thankfully one I didn't use elsewhere) for a website and assured me he knew I'd used the password to access a porn site and promised that unless I paid huge sums in Bitcoin he would release footage taken through my webcam of me watching the porn. Since I'd accessed no porn site and the password was useless there was no practical reason to worry, but it felt like the negative energy levels of the world were rising. I was tired from travelling, I was hormonal and I was working hard at all the things that work to raise my mood – choosing to have a good day; practising gratitude; calling up what Tara Mohr calls your Inner Mentor; being mindful; bingeing on sugar…

And would my visit to Douglas help? It seemed unlikely from what I'd read – I was leaving sleepy Sunset City for the town that was the headquarters of the world's largest online poker company. And I remembered what the taxi driver had said about the drug problem. Since this represented all that I knew about the island's capital, it didn't suggest much soul.

The route to get there took us through estates of meanly proportioned houses. We passed a tiny garden where a little girl, perhaps aged four, ran furiously and pointlessly round and round like a goldfish in a bowl. Or like an islander looking for a way out? Or like the negative energy in my grumpy head.

We passed Tynwald Hill – home of what is claimed to be the world's longest unbroken parliamentary tradition. Long before experiments such as the Brahma Kumaris all-female leadership (it is now the largest women-run faith organisation in the world), this was a place where over a thousand years ago the Vikings established a place of assembly. The steep-sided hill seemed surprisingly small but talking about the island's democratic traditions with one of the shopkeepers in Peel he had suggested that you could have too much democracy. There are twenty-four districts on the island and each one has a commissioner. There are also twenty-four Members of the House of Keys (MHKs – whose roles are like that of British MPs), and a district like Peel's, with just six thousand registered electors, returns two MHKs. In addition, on the annual Tynwald Day, any Isle of Man citizen can present their proposal to the island's parliament. It's an extraordinary level of representation – or of cumbersome bureaucracy, depending on your point of view. Perhaps it's a good thing not to build the sides of your parliamentary site too shallow.

Eventually we arrived in Douglas. It was a long way from the Las Vegas I had imagined for the headquarters of online poker. We walked along the om-pom-promenade, passing slow trams drawn by jingling horses; the air was sluggish with nostalgia. Heading north out of town took you onto the headland beyond the Hollywood-style letters set into the hillside spelling out ELECTRIC RAILWAY. The houses here were clearly built for retirement – not places to accommodate full families, to bring up children. These were places focused on the need for *sun*, the need to *lounge*. With their glassed frontages they were built on an architecture of maximising small pleasures. I found them good reminders of mindfulness.

From here I could look down at the neo-Gothic Tower of Refuge built on rocks which had claimed many lives in Douglas Bay. The tower was the idea of Manxman Sir William Hillary, the founder of the RNLI; the concept of his island as a place of rescue and refuge was growing on me.

Down again on the sea front I ate battered-and-deep-fried 'Manx Queenie' scallops out of a paper cone and strolled until the municipal marigolds ran out. At that point I caught a taxi to get to the Brahma Kumaris.

The centre is housed within a flat in a small modern housing estate, though Gill, from the BK community here, later told me that she estimated that ten per cent of the island's population had been through the doors of this modest place at some point. I rang the bell and Joanna came to greet me. I was early but she said they had just finished eating. There was a strong smell of something spicy which surprised me as one of the things I had learned about the Brahma Kumaris was that their vegetarian diet excluded onions and garlic. Later, BKs told me about how you could use the dried gum, asafoetida, as a substitute and about the BK approach to eating as a meditative experience which is done mindfully rather than while you talk or read.

Joanna smiled in welcome with the open face, unfurrowed brow and beautiful skin of a nun. I never did find out about her family situation but, along with vegetarianism, another of the BK community's tenets is celibacy. She chuckled when I asked her about it later – 'Yes, it's not for everyone.' The word 'kumari' itself means an unmarried woman and although Brahma Kumaris was founded by a man, he set up a council of women to run the organisation and following his death it has been entirely led by women.

I had been expecting (perhaps ironically on this Isle of Man) to find an oestrogen-rich atmosphere here but to my surprise Joanna told me that 'the other course participant hasn't arrived yet, but he'll be here soon.'

'Er... *he*?'

Brian was one of several men who've been involved with the BK here for a while. He works for a company offering financial services – like one fifth of the workforce on Man who are employed in insurance, banking, accountancy and business and corporate services. As an offshore company, his employer would pay no local taxes on capital growth.

But it's always better to meet people than to read their company's websites – Brian's sincerity shone through his stories of how he'd looked for inner peace in travels that had taken him in the last twenty years around the world and through many of the pages of the Reader's Digest *Guide to World Religions*. He was echoed by Gill, to whom I spoke afterwards, as one of the first to start attending BK activities on the island. Now seventy-four, she described having sampled a range of alternative groups ('I tried the Buddhist group but I found them a bit soulless'?) before landing with BK.

These pilgrims – these faith tourists – and their routes intrigued me as much as this group they had ended up in. Joanna told me 'there's a woman who comes here and says that she is a Christian but for her spirituality she has to look beyond the church.' Joanna herself is ecumenical in her approach: 'All the religions have the same message; that we're spiritual beings on a journey to the light – but the older religions have so much sociocultural stuff layered on top of it that it's become distorted.' I remembered my parallel experiences at Peterborough's Hindu mandir and its churches.

Later I spoke to Anthony who has been a member of the BK community here since 2001. He held a lay position in his local church, but says 'Anglican silences are not silences at all. They have in the service something that says "a period of reflective silence" but they charge on as quickly as they can.'

So did Brian consider this a religion? A way of life?

'It's a good way to relax. I used to walk a lot but now I have a problem with my leg so this is good for me. You feel refreshed and tranquil; you're more tolerant and focused. In a word, what it's given me is peace.'

I thought about some of the other World Religions and what they demanded of their followers, and found it inspiring to be in a place of religion that's like a good long walk. I remembered the BK mission statement – a spiritual movement 'dedicated to personal transformation and world renewal'. Later Joanna wrote out for us, *When I change, the world changes*; Brian was doing his bit.

I asked what his colleagues thought of him coming here, and he twisted his face unmeditatively, 'I work in IT,' he said as if this was an explanation. 'So I wouldn't really mention it to the guys.'

Brian and I took our seats in a rather John Lennon room – cream-coloured walls, carpet, curtains, furniture and flipchart. Joanna herself was all in white. The setting made the splashes of colour in the room all the more striking. There was an orange picture dominating the room, an abstract sunburst which I recognised as a reworking of the BK symbol. There was an orange rock-salt lamp and orange chrysanthemums. And there was us and the silence.

The flip chart at least started to fill up as Joanna recapped the previous course sessions, which Brian had attended. The Raja yoga meditation course is just one of the activities run here – there are weekly meet-ups, a daily 6.30am meditation and one-off courses on well-being, on the power of positive thinking, on wholesome eating. I mused that it seemed less like a Reader's Digest-certified World Religion than a Personal Health and Social Education curriculum.

Perhaps I was disappointed, but it certainly made the learning here easier to absorb. The flip chart's messages were simple, mainly unsurprising, but no less powerful for that.

We can choose who we are; our identity doesn't need to be affected by external things – by how our hair looks today, our success at work. Yes, that attempted blackmailer could only be present in my thoughts as much as I wanted him to be. Later, another of the community who told me the biggest impact the centre and its teachings had on her over the last twenty years, amplified this – 'No-one can take away your happiness unless you give them permission; I have the capacity to be joyful regardless of my circumstances.' They're startling truths that I can see could be life-changing.

Love, happiness and peace need to come from inside, not from temporary things. I thought reluctantly of the deep-fried queenie scallops in their mayonnaise dressing – there had been happiness there. I thought about youth and ageing, but of course I knew that fundamentally this statement about love, happiness and peace was true.

We can use affirmations, in the present and the positive. Joanna suggested 'I love and accept myself', or 'I live in the present moment'. My nagging wrong-side-of-bed feelings this morning ought to be easily conquerable – I considered a repeated phrase to replace that kid tearing up my gardens as she trundled destructively round and round in my head. I thought back to the four-year-old and in my mind I made her skip, as if this happiness business could be as easy as flipping a switch.

We can do daily tasks with love. Joanna talked about the drudgery of housework, of meal preparation for others, and how it can be transformed with what she called 'karma yoga', and Brian talked about having tried to take this approach to ironing. I loved the idea but I struggled to think of a chance to practise it. I don't iron. Rob cleans the house when it needs it badly enough and we have a cleaner who comes on the rare occasions when we conclude (usually because we're about to have guests) that more should be done. Rob and I generally make our own meals, me eating at lunchtime when I'm home and he in the evening. To be more yogic was I actually going to have to do more housework?

From there the course got harder: *When the body dies there's something that lives.* We were well beyond the PSHE curriculum now, and beyond my own belief system – that nothing survives our death, or if there is then it is only the impact of our actions.

The soul's original qualities are peace, love, happiness, purity, power, wisdom. And the soul resides in the centre of the forehead. Now I was lost.

Joanna went on to talk about karma (she pronounced the R). She said that if there's someone you get on with then it is possible that you have 'karmic credits' with them because your souls have had contact before, and I started to feel cross. This was a fairy tale, surely?

Brian joined in with how he understands karma – 'Well, it's nice to be nice and you get the benefit straight away because it feels good to be nice'. You couldn't argue with that, and I breathed.

Which was appropriate because now we were going to do some meditation. Joanna suggested that we used the time to be taken back to who we were, intrinsically; to 'connect with the source of light'. She likened it to sunbathing and I imagined myself unfurling like a daisy.

She suggested meditating on this source of light with our eyes open, which is my favourite kind of meditation at home, though I've always suspected that's because it gives me something to *do* when psychic boredom kicks in. I know this is not supposed to be the purpose, and I try not to let my eyes stray from the candle or landscape or flower or whatever I have chosen to focus on. Here I'd have others to hold me accountable so I prepared to try very hard.

Joanna reminded us of the things that could disturb the mind when we sat down to meditate: attachment (to people); self-gratification (meaning the sources of our gratification through the instant pleasures through the senses – it is true that with embarrassing frequency I interrupt my meditations with thoughts of what my next meal will be); the ego ('trying to take our estimation of self-worth from a temporary and limited self-image'); and anger, which she identified as being a feeling of frustration when any of the other three behaviours are threatened. I remembered the email from my colleague. Of course the explanation of how I'd messed up had threatened my carefully constructed 'limited self-image' (of my professional perfection).

There was a settling silence as would have been approved by that 1904 guidebook. Here was the resting-place for the toil-worn worker from the hurrying outer world.

I'd been meditating for a few years now and had started to develop my own principles for my daily practice. Yes, I should be still, which means no fidgeting or scratching; in one particularly 'enlightened' session I even allowed a mosquito to bite me in six different places rather than lose my focus. I was proud of that. However, unlike some meditation disciplines, I allowed myself to shift and readjust when I felt pins and needles on the way. And I tried to take as much of the ritual out of my practice. I don't understand – perhaps haven't yet learned – the importance of physical symmetry for meditation that some schools teach as so important: I feel that I can access my subconscious whether I'm on a park bench or a special cushion. I often end up doing my meditation on public transport for example, so I'm not used to creating special spaces or poses in order to start. I just seat myself as if I'm about to settle for a good catch-up with an old friend. Which, in a way, I am. I don't chant (I only tried that once, as a way of keeping myself awake, but it was like the time I tried karaoke – a horrible drone which interfered with the music, and which it took me some time to realise was me) and I make no special mudra with my fingers.

Here, I had one leg casually crossed over the other. Joanna said we were ready to begin. There was a pause. Then she said:

'Er, you've done meditation before, Elizabeth, right?'

I wasn't symmetrical. I wasn't, as Caroline at Brimham Rocks would have it, sitting as if I was about to do something special. Obediently, I uncrossed my legs and Joanna finally pressed 'play'.

The meditation had what was called a 'commentary'; layered over plinky-plonky music an Indian voice directed what we should be thinking about. When I had first started meditation I'd tried various such recordings as downloads from the internet, but it wasn't long before, inexpert as I was, I just wanted the voices to be quiet. I was trying *not* to think. I had the same difficulties with this man. Eventually he announced 'and now we will have a moment of peace'.

But I could feel it coming, with a physiological panic. Perhaps it was the chrysanthemums but I was… going… to … *sneeze*!

It shattered any moment of peace any of us might have been having.

I tensed in embarrassment. There was a more profound silence after my great spluttering interruption, and I decided it would probably make it worse if I said something to apologise.

Everyone was too polite afterwards to mention my explosion of our shared moment of peace but it did raise a question I'd been grappling with ever since I started practising daily meditation. The BK leaflet I was given for 'simple meditation practice' fitted with advice and direction that others had given me. 'Become aware of all sounds around you, be in the present' it said. It also said 'follow your breathing'. In my experience it's impossible to do both. Either you're being mindful (I do believe this makes you happy; I'm sure it makes you a better writer) – noticing and savouring all the sounds, smells, sensations and sights around you – or you're focusing on the breath. After experimenting, my own conclusion is that I try to be mindful when I'm in the rest of my life – when I'm sitting at table, when I'm on the bus, when I'm walking down the street. But when I'm meditating it's time to be mind*less*; time to focus only on the breath.

Thinking about any of this is of course a disaster for effective meditation of either kind.

Nevertheless, after this session of meditation and meta-meditation I could feel my mind settled. The little girl was no longer racing round the tiny garden. Perhaps she had even stopped occasionally to pick some flowers. When there was more discussion I kept quiet again, and calm, about my views on karma. We finished the session with another meditation, this time guided by a woman's voice.

Leaving the centre I could feel the familiar blissed-out state keeping me not just 'relaxed' (a word that we don't use correctly. After all, if we really – really – relaxed we'd become something between a baby and a corpse, sphincters released, heart not beating, digestion halted). But I felt *still*.

Speaking afterwards to other members of the BK community on Man, they talked about a similar impact of being part of the community. 'It takes away any fear – you know the story, you know where you're coming from, you know where you're going.' Gill said, 'Psychologists say our biggest fear is death but I don't fear death.' *Traa dy liooar* indeed. Anthony talked about the tools he'd gained for dealing with his depression, and how he'd been liberated from that, as well as from the fear of it which 'is as bad as the depression'.

Gill added that coming together with others who have that same certainty and freedom was part of what attracts her to the group. 'There is a feeling of light when you see these people, they're on your wavelength.' Anthony went further, identifying the BK community that he feels part of which transcends the community on the island. He's met BK community members from Portugal and Spain who'd come to Man. I was lucky to have been given a chance to glimpse it.

Night was falling across the island as I was driven back to Douglas; a dark night when I knew I would be able to see far-off stars if I tried. And despite the TT race and the other, deep-fried, pleasures of instant gratification along the promenade, perhaps it was true that there was something special about the island's call to spirituality and what Sue, from the BKs, had described as its 'positive energy'.

Joanna had been practical about it when I'd asked her – she'd pointed out that when the Isle of Man BK group had started in 1994 it was the only group on the island offering spiritual courses. 'And when you want something on an island you can't just go on looking in the next town.' So the isolation that had created a niche for the genes for tailless cats here had perhaps also created the niche for another minority community to flourish.

But, unlike the others on this island, I could just go on looking in the next town – because the next morning I was off. Which meant I was onto the ferry, and I was inhaling diesel while my stomach sloshed like bilge water. And I'd be trapped in this swaying state for four hours. I could feel my shoulders hunching, my jaw setting and the behaviours my doctor friend calls 'voluntary guarding' in abdominal anticipation of a painful experience.

I was sad to be on my way – leaving an island has something final about it; it's not just like your train pulling out of Peterborough. Sitting in one of the few seats left when I'd got into the ferry's saloon, by the toilets and with no view of the horizon to help me orient, I closed my eyes and listened to the graunches and rattles as the engine started up, chains rang out and the passengers gave a collective shudder. It wasn't going to be a smooth crossing. I stopped listening and turned my focus inward. I even uncrossed my legs. If you're feeling seasick, go down into the engine room.

Gratitude diary entry
Rob's full head of hair – and that he had not become bald
by thirty as he'd warned me would happen when we met,
aged nineteen

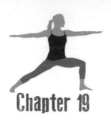

Chapter 19

Pranayama – Liverpool

'Pay it forward'

Any yoga journey around Britain has an important stop in the hometown of the four musicians who gave yoga its cool. While Iyengar's yoga may have captured the hearts and headstands of north London's upper-middle classes and ILEA's evening classes, it wasn't until the Beatles's well-publicised experimentations and stay on an ashram in Rishikesh that the Carnaby Street set were interested.

It was while the Fab Four were filming *Help!* in 1965 that they met Swami Vishnudevananda, the founder of Sivananda yoga. He presented them with signed copies of his work, *The Complete Illustrated Book of Yoga*, which was, for George Harrison in particular, the starting point for a study of yoga and Eastern religion. Their explorations eventually took the group to Rishikesh and to learn Transcendental Meditation.

The faces of the four lads smiled down at me from the wall of my Airbnb room. They smiled from the souvenir shops and adverts all around Liverpool, too. They sang to me at every opportunity, snatches of their melodies and lyrics escaping every time a tour bus went past or the doors swung open in a shop aimed at the city's visitors.

'Oh, I get by with a little help from my friends, with a little help from my …'

I had come to Liverpool to study a particular approach to yoga: the focus on breathing which may be the only common thread running through the schools of yoga. From the fourth-century yoga sutras of Patanjali through the fifteenth-century Hatha yoga Pradipika and the twentieth-century works of Krishnamacharya and his disciples, Jois and Iyengar; whether yoga is seen as a primarily spiritual discipline or a primarily physical one, the attention to one's breathing is shared by all these complementary and sometimes conflicting ways of using yoga. And to explore what 'pranayama' – the practice of the breath – might be like I had chosen to come to Liverpool as the town in Britain most buffeted by breath; the UK's windiest city.

However, I found myself here on a still day. I checked the unintended poetry of the Beaufort Wind Scale:

0:   sea like a mirror
     smoke rises vertically
1:   ripples with appearance of scales are formed, without
     foam crests direction shown by smoke drift
2:   crests have a glassy appearance but do not break
     leaves rustle
3:   scattered white horses
     leaves and small twigs in constant motion
4:   raises dust
5:   chance of some spray
     small trees in leaf begin to sway
6:   umbrellas used with difficulty
7:   spindrift begins to be seen
     whole trees in motion
8:   impedes progress
9:   spray affects visibility
     chimney pots and slates removed

10: trees uprooted

11: medium-sized ships for a long time lost to view behind the waves

12: the air is filled with foam and spray

Devastation

We were at zero – smoke rose vertically: there was no wind at all. Indeed, everything seemed to have stopped, with chaos on the trains so that my connection arrived late to get the replacement bus service. I asked the bus driver what time he thought we'd get to my final stop, near Liverpool Hope University, and whether I'd then be able to get a taxi to the yoga class so I wouldn't miss the beginning. It was going to be tight.

The bus crawled through the suburbs of Liverpool, giving me time to stare out at them and muse. I wanted to know more about where the names came from – Court Hey Park. Alder Hey, Huyton Hey… They sounded jaunty.

Then the bus came to a halt. People got up to leave and one man who'd obviously overheard me talking to the driver said, 'This is your stop. But you know, I don't think you'll get a taxi from here – there's no rank.'

Without a taxi there was no way I'd get to the class on time. I may have looked unyogically panicked.

'Will there be a minicab office nearby?'

A woman standing in the queue waiting to get off the bus answered me,

'I can drive you; it's not far.'

It seemed an extraordinary thing to offer. And I wondered what the catch might be; was it safe?

'Are you going that way?' I asked.

'Not really, but it will only be ten minutes.'

'You wouldn't get that in the south,' I quipped but Trish explained that she was in fact from the south. She'd been in Liverpool for sixteen years, though; perhaps that accounted for it.

I wondered, and continued to wonder as we got into her car and as she typed into her satnav the postcode I gave her and as she drove me away: what prompted her to add this detour to the end of her working day? Why are we kind?

Trish told me she worked as a psychotherapist for a charity called Freedom from Torture. It's not as if she needed to atone for anything then; it's not as if she hadn't already spent her day doing good, and giving to those in need. I started to feel almost guilty that I was using up her supplies when there were others in her care who needed her generosity so much more.

On our journey I told her a bit about why I was visiting Liverpool and this yoga class, and she told me about the yoga classes offered for the survivors of torture she worked with in Manchester.

When she dropped me at the entrance to Hope University I wondered if I should offer to pay her petrol money. Or would that be offensive? I blurted out yet more thanks.

'And, I'll... I'll pay it forward,' I promised. It was quite a commitment.

I made it to the class just in time.

... I get by with a little help from my friends.

The room was darkened and still, with the other twenty or so yogis and yoginis already poised on their mats when I entered. I hurried to settle myself, but looking round I realised that there was no supply of class mats here.

I had learned that your mat is supposed to be an area that is both practical, for orientation ('move to the front of your mat'), and conceptual. It marks out your space – and ensures that you don't hit someone in the face in an overenthusiastic Warrior pose. Yoga websites and magazines give reviews of the latest mats, of those with antibacterial properties, those that are cushioned or 'grippy', sweat-resistant, printed with alignment lines, recyclable or made from natural tree rubber for a truly enlightened practice. The best retail at over a hundred pounds. But I've failed to get fetishistic about my mat. I had enough to cope with managing transport of my rucksack around the country, so I was happy to take whatever was offered to me in the public classes I attended. In my home practice I actively preferred the process of transforming any space into a sacred space without needing a vinyl rectangle to do it.

However, now I was in a dusty university conference room with nothing to place between my bare toes and the patchily sticky carpet tile. Creating a sacred space seemed a bit more challenging under such circumstances.

Luckily I had in my bag what I always have in my bag. There are five things I won't travel without. One is Febreze (useful in uncertain Airbnb accommodation and where washing machines are scarce on the road). Another is a decent teabag – meaning any kettle, primus stove or samovar can quickly produce a reassuring warm drink of familiar taste and health benefits (my teabag is usually green) to be cradled between palms and raised with fragrant steam in a small private ritual of celebration. Then there's duct tape, for holding anything together – mending broken shoes, improvising suitcases from rice sacks, or sealing half-finished packs of crisps to be eaten later. I've even been known to whip it out to keep down health-and-safety-hazard errant carpet spotted at the top of stairs on my travels. I have yet to use it to hold together the edges of a wound until I can receive medical attention but it pleases me to know I could.

I always have with me my flask as well – for the tea or for water so as to save single-use plastic water bottles. And I also always have an Indian cotton bedspread.

The bedspread has been a friend on picnics, a towel after impromptu bathing, a sunburn cover-up, an aeroplane pillow, a wrap to enable me to enter mosques when I was caught with bare arms, or an extra layer of bedlinen in cold hostels. Tonight in Liverpool, for the first time it became a yoga mat.

I folded it in quarters and sat comfortably down and looked at my fellow practitioners. The class was typical of the other yoga groups I'd met so far – about twenty people, of whom three were men. The average age was older here though – I was one of the youngest, and definitely one of the more fit. Liverpool is a city with health challenges – significantly higher levels of smoking than the national rate, apparently also with significantly lower rates of people eating their 'five a day'. Hospital admissions for alcohol-specific conditions in the city are almost three times the national average, and there's a rate of death from drug misuse that's twice the national rate. Most shockingly, and obviously not relevant to this class, around twenty-five per cent of adults are physically inactive, meaning they spend fewer than thirty minutes a week on moderately intense exercise. It was good to be reminded, with all the overthinking that's possible in a yoga class about holding a position correctly or synchronising breath appropriately, how just moving your body around for an hour's class a week brings benefits. It's what those adult education course designers knew in London in the 1960s; that this is a public good as well as potentially a private spiritual journey.

Rosemary – or Prema – was now opening the class. Her spiritual name was given to her by her teacher, and I learned later means 'Divine Love'. She explained when we discussed it that the idea of being given a name is to reflect the qualities of the individual but also to help them grow spiritually. She showed plenty of love tonight.

With a sweet little-girl voice she reminded us of the inhale or exhale for each movement, and led us in a standard Cat and Cow warm-up which always exquisitely loosens the lower back, in just the place it seems to seize up. I added the trick I'd been taught in one of my first yoga sessions of what I liked to call 'Curious Cow', so that as my back arched concave, head and butt in the air, I turned my head to gaze bovinely at my right and left rumps in turn. It was the perfect way to loosen up after my multiple forms of transport today and their associated tensions.

Then, from lying on our backs Prema invited us to roll back and forth, 'a massage for the derriere' as she put it, lapsing out of Sanskrit terminology briefly.

The class had a down-to-earth atmosphere that I'd missed in my fancier wanderings since Port Isaac. If you're holding positions like Warrior or Triangle you get a good view of the ceiling in a yoga class. The Iyengar Institute had thought this through with its skylights; the Hope University Conference Centre had not. I looked up at smoke detectors, sprinkler systems, a projector and strip lighting. Around us was a clutter of stacked chairs and flipchart stands, less acrobatic than their name might suggest. This is the reality for most people who do yoga in Britain; not Lululemon or the indulgence of day-long workshops in Stroud, but a quick class somewhere near to home in a venue that doubles up for other purposes during the day.

From Downward-facing Dog we moved our right leg into lunge (I did it in one. This does not always happen) and then positioned the right hand to be on the left-hand side of the leg.

'Feel how the arm and the leg support one another, working against one another,' Prema prompted us. I had lost count of the number of ways that the word 'yoga' had been explained to me. Everyone agreed that it came from the same Indo-European root as 'yoke' and signified a joining up. But what was being joined to what? Some people said it was body and soul. Some said it was individual with the Absolute. Tonight we were focused on the connection between body and breath (which, as 'spirit', might be the same as the first explanation). But here Prema was showing how joining our bodies up with themselves could be a source of strength and balance. A good yoga class reminds me of my three dimensions, even without worrying about the fourth. Even the simplest pose of Cobbler, sitting with the bottoms of your feet against one another, can be for me a startling chance for the soles (if not the souls) to feel and be felt. These are the things that yoga can do to join you up.

But here, under Prema's guidance, with each pose we focused not only on the muscles and the shape we were making, but on that *prana* that flowed through us. Prema reminded us how the *in* breath was nourishing, the *out* breath cleansing.

From standing we came back down to our mats, the room crackling like wildfire as forty knees flexed. I still can't believe that this sound is actually caused by small air bubbles in the synaptic fluid – that we are popping some internal bladderwrack or bubblewrap as we bend. We were taken into a shoulder stand and then out into Plough. In case we lost our way in all these moves, Prema had provided a beautiful stick-figure diagram of the class plan which was available for everyone to have with them and take away. The A4 sheets were covered with tiny creatures flexing and writhing, standing up and stretching out on the ground. I counted ninety-two exquisite little figures on one side of the page. It was like a cave painting of an orgy, or a battlefield.

In fact what it most reminded me of was the drawings in my Good News Bible as a child. The attitudes of praise, the zest of the illustration for Deuteronomy's 'Choose life!' verse that I remembered from decades ago matched exactly the upward fling of arms in Dancer pose. I'd never seen such a lovely way of capturing a session.

We reached the end of the figures and the road map they had offered, and now we did some focused prana work, sitting up and creating a *dhyana* mudra, holding one cupped hand in the cup of the other and touching the thumb tips together as we breathed. Then we made what I learned was called a Vishnu mudra, holding the little finger and ring finger down and with the two other fingers and thumb closing alternating nostrils. I find pranayama exercises like this tough. I guess, being honest, I find them boring. But I know you have to learn ways of noticing and being conscious of the breath. I thought of all the times I had used what yoga had taught me about the breath; of standing in the wings of the stage before I made my speech at a huge conference, and reducing the glare of the scary world to *in* and *out*; of arguments and heartache that had been warded off or softened, by turning my awareness to those draughts of cooling air coursing down my throat, the literal inspiration that was available to me twelve times a minute.

Eventually, with many a 'ta-raa' the class broke up and I headed to the train.

Once I'd got a seat I started to write up some of my notes on my laptop. The woman next to me was discreetly stretching her neck to try to see what I was typing.

'Do you work in Liverpool?' she asked. She pronounced it 'wairk'.

I told her about having come to try yoga here. She was a generation older than me, now slumped in her seat and smoothing her hands over a belly that bulged above her waistband. I remembered the city's health statistics. I was sure she'd have heard of yoga, but I decided not to explain the specifics of pranayama.

'Oh yes, I started yoga classes because of my next-door neighbour. I thought it would be hard because of my osteoarthritis, but after three sessions I stopped taking all my pills. But why Liverpool?' she asked and had never heard that it was Britain's windiest city – though you couldn't always believe statistics, I mused, thinking not only about the weather today but about my preconceptions of her.

'Ha, I can say this because I'm Liverpool born and bred,' she snickered. 'But if Liverpool's Britain's windiest city, that's just the people!

'But that yoga breathing is how I get to sleep at night. My yoga teacher was pregnant at the same time as my daughter but she managed to have her baby with no drugs – just using yoga breathing.

'My other daughter's got a little bit weighty and I've been telling her to do yoga. I recommend it to everyone.'

It was another form of passing it on, of paying it forward, a final reminder as the train left the station, of the currents that can blow from Liverpool around the world:

…a little help from my frieeeeeends!

Gratitude diary entry
waking to an email from someone wanting to help with my idea for a social enterprise

Chapter 20

Laughter Yoga – Blackpool

'Oh ho haaa ha ha ha ha ha!'

The air smelt sugary. And fried. Like doughnuts, or candyfloss, or toffee apples. Like transgression, like instant gratification; this was kiss-me-quick nutrition.

I had arrived in out-of-season Blackpool to try a session of Laughter Yoga. This was Blackpool even out of party-conference-season; there were no parties here. It was raining.

The weather was so bad that the top of the iconic 158m tower was shrouded in mist. Nevertheless, even being able to see the base was enough to tell you that you had arrived on holiday. Like its older brother on Paris's Champ de Mars, the structure is designed to dominate the city's skyline; it defines the Blackpool brand. It may also have been designed to make you believe you were in Paris – if you'd never been to Paris.

As the clouds swirled around the tower's tip, every so often a flag could be glimpsed up there, defiantly triumphant. Blackpool will remain upbeat, whatever the conditions. All around me, signs reminded me of that – *Kids Eat Free*! *Amusements*! *Funland*! *Jackpot*! Even the pool of sick I stepped over on the pavement was pink.

I'd arrived on an overnight bus after days of travelling. Before going to the Laughter Yoga session I badly needed breakfast – I reviewed my consumption and realised that over the preceding three days all I'd had to eat were some vegan biscuits, an aeroplane snack-size bag of pretzels, a packet of crisps, a turmeric latte, some bowls of cereal, a forkful of potatoes snatched from a pan on the hob in my friend's house where I'd stopped off en route, and a glass of wine. With the exception of two snack-pots of pureed fruit, there had been no vitamins. I seriously needed nutrients.

I passed a shop selling sticks of prosecco-flavoured rock.

I was finding this a barren place. And slightly eerie. A 'joke shop' advertised that it sold air rifles and masks, which seemed less like comedy than equipping a light terrorist group.

I remembered the footage I'd seen of the town's iconic Laughing Man: a clown in a glass box laughing maniacally and endlessly at the passers-by, rocking as he did so. *Oh ho haaaa ha ha ha ha ha! Oh ho haaaa ha ha ha ha ha! Oh ho haaaa ha ha ha ha ha!* ... Like the end of a horror film, the clown burned up in the Blackpool Pleasure Beach fire a few years ago, and as I crossed the road from the 'joke shop' I imagined the clown's silken outfit turning sticky, his orange wig melting in the flames, his voice slurring until he expired on a final faint *haaaa*.

With hunger driving me to ever more disturbing hallucinations, the Palma Café appeared like a beacon. It proudly announced that it was established in 1965, and the condensation on the windows suggested it was warm inside, so I went in. There were leatherette banquettes the greyed-green colour of the sea today, and at each was a Formica table with a plastic cruet set of a vinegar bottle and an enormous salt shaker that could have doubled as a flour dredger. I guessed that here you could get chips with everything. Like the rest of the town, it was almost deserted, though a mum, grandma and baby sat at one table and at another were a couple of pensioners. I sank gratefully into a banquette and ordered the only vitamins I could see on the menu, in the form of a veggie burger.

What did I want to drink?

I flipped through the menu. The Blackpool feeling was getting to me and I felt ready for Amusements and Jackpot and surprising bonuses. As one of the women I met in the town said later, 'Coachloads who come to the seaside: they're up for anything.'

Within my limits I was up for anything, and when I saw Dr Pepper listed I thought I'd try something new. Someone once told me it was like drinking lemonade when you have Germolene on your lips.

At the first sip I remembered that they've stopped making the old pink Germolene, and I wondered whether this was because people complained of the taste it gave things after you put it on your lips: I found Dr Pepper truly revolting.

I went up to the counter and asked for something different. Comforting after a restless night among strangers; warming on a day of rain. Some national nostalgia inspired by the Victorian tower, or some personal nostalgia for childhood comforts, and remembering the promise of Slough's most famous product, I ordered one of those mugs of Horlicks that gives 'fitness and stamina that prevents undue fatigue'.

Just as the advert promised, with every sip I started to revive, and I tuned in to the conversations of those around me.

'Are you watching t'fireworks?' one of the old men asked the other. Looking at the drizzle out of the window, anything taking place this evening seemed likely to be a display of damp squibs, but I raised my Horlicks in a toast to Blackpool's eternal optimism.

After my unorthodox breakfast I still had time before the Laughter Yoga session, and online I'd found a gym where I could get a day pass. In my experiences of travel by night bus since my bleary experiences in Edinburgh this was one of the hacks I'd come to find most useful

– when you arrive in a town with heavy luggage and the grunge of a night half-asleep in diesel fumes, you have the option of getting a hostel, just to use the shower and stow your stuff, with the full price of a night's accommodation, or you can pay the often exorbitant cost of left luggage (in London that can easily be a tenner) with no shower. Or you can buy a £4.50 day-pass at a gym and get use of a locker for the day and use of a shower. If you want – but you don't have to – you can even use a running machine. I like using this little trick on my travels because it makes me feel like Jack Reacher.

In the changing room, the rucksack was, as always, a good ice-breaker. (I imagine this is not just a metaphor – it was heavy enough today that it could have been hurled anywhere in the Arctic and opened up an immediate fishing hole.) The woman watching the logistics of unpacking and repacking asked me conversationally where I was going, so I explained about my yoga journey around Britain. Yoga is as good an icebreaker as a rucksack (and far more portable), and as she and I each quietly struggled with straps and elastics she told me about the yoga sessions held at this gym, and we were soon talking about life-changing stuff that you don't often get into with a stranger within a few minutes of meeting. Especially when you're in your underwear.

Having exercised, showered and dressed in clean clothes, I made my way to the venue where I'd been told that a group of Laughter Yoga leaders was being trained. There was no reception desk and as I wandered through fire doors in anonymous corridors in search of the course, it was only when I heard the sound of giggling from one of the rooms that I knew I'd found it.

The five women here were being trained to be able to lead some of the more than one hundred Laughter Clubs that have been set up around the UK over the last ten years. Their trainer was Lotte and when I pushed open the door I found her chortling to an appreciative audience.

'Ho ho ho ho ho!' she went, and

'Ho ho ho ho ho!' replied her group.

I smiled politely, and Lotte stopped to introduce me and to explain what they were doing. This was the second day of these Laughter Yoga leaders' training, and for the purposes of the training, Lotte had already established with the group that when she gave a laugh, they had to copy. It led to behaviour that seemed bizarrely sycophantic, when the teacher gave a fake laugh (she called it 'unconditional laughter') and then the whole group mimicked it.

'I was explaining,' said Lotte, 'that there's a difference between ho-ho-ho laughs, which are from the belly, and ha-ha-ha laughs, which come from your centre, and he-he-he laughs which come from your chest or throat and are superficial. If you repeat this kind for too long you can damage your larynx.'

I felt like I did when I first started yoga and learned about breathing, and how something I'd taken for granted was more complicated, and more important, than I had ever realised; I was Monsieur Jordain discovering that he's been speaking prose all his life.

'We call this Laughter *Yoga*,' Lotte went on, 'because it combines deep-breathing techniques with laughter. Social laughter lasts from three to five seconds and is shallow; just generated in the chest. But Laughter Yoga prepares you to do ten to fifteen minutes of laughter to reap the physical benefits of laughter that engages the diaphragm.'

Ten to fifteen minutes! It seemed a lot of laughter, even though I knew from my reading that I was thankfully not going to be expected to wait until I actually found anything funny before I laughed. The founder of Laughter Yoga, Dr Madan Kataria, says that at first when he got people together he brought a selection of jokes to 'make' them laugh. As the joke supply ran out, the jokes people shared became increasingly risqué and sometimes hurtful. The movement was in crisis until he discovered that our bodies can't tell the difference between faked laughter and real. Thus saved from hours of knock-knock, people started to feel like smiling, so today would be about forced, 'unconditional' laughter as a regime.

'But people still find it hard to find ways of laughing for that long each day,' Lotte said, 'so that's why we've started our Laughter Yoga telephone call every day. You can dial in every morning to laugh with about ten other people.'

Lotte continued with her deadpan taxonomy of laughter: the shoulder-shaking laugh and silent laughter, and then the chemical implications of laughing. 'Laughter is powerful. It increases blood supply, and that's why I don't like people doing Laughter Yoga when they've had alcohol as it pushes the alcohol round the system faster and gives it greater impact on the body.

'Laughter also produces dopamine and endorphins,' she said. 'Endorphins boost the immune system, and this is how I got into Laughter Yoga, because I was diagnosed with MS and knew my immune system was weak.'

Suddenly the fake laughter didn't sound quite so silly; it sounded rather courageous.

We began our laughter exercises, using techniques Lotte has refined during her years of training: she reckons she's trained over a thousand Laughter Club leaders, and now does two or three corporate Laughter Yoga sessions a week. We started with speeding up our laughter, at first giving a slow, unconvincing (unconvinced) laugh that we took up to chuckle before breaking into a full titter. In early riding lessons I remember learning the names for the pacing of horses – from *trot* to *canter* and on. Soon we were all positively galloping through ecstatic peals of laughter.

There's a practical problem here that will be spotted by any teacher who's led PE for an excited group of primary school pupils. How do you get their attention back when you've just set them off on an all-absorbing and high-volume activity? Lotte had thought this through and the group had already established a tribal call:

'Very good! Very good! YAY!' Lotte called enthusiastically, clapping once on each of the 'very's and raising her hands in celebration on the 'yay!'.

Obediently the group stopped laughing and repeated in time:

'Very good! Very good! YAY!'

Throughout the day the call was used to bring us to order or to break up discussion, punctuating the session like 'Amen' or 'Allelujah' at a religious revival.

Then we did an exercise which paired us off and where we gave our partner a handshake, first with one hand, then with the other. Then holding both hands as if we were country dancing, we spun each other around, giggling all the time. Next Lotte described a little scenario where we had to imagine preparing to go on holiday, getting out our passport from the drawer and laughing at the photo of ourselves that we find there. We all mimed the scene, as well as the following one where we arrived on holiday in Hawaii and were greeted 'Aloha-ha-ha' – our hands waved up and then rained down on the 'ha ha ha'. We bowed 'namaste' to one another with hands in prayer position to each person while doing what I'd call chuckling.

With the increased laughter I was doing I was feeling very self-conscious. Like saying a word over and over until it loses all meaning and seems ridiculous, the repeated guffawing didn't feel funny; it felt animal. I started to notice how it also sounded a lot like orgasm.

I was also reminded of a feature of my laugh that I had been teased about as a teenager – the self-deprecating or embarrassed inhalation hissed under my tongue at the sides of my mouth almost as if I'm trying to suck back the fountain of mirth that had just sprayed (hopefully not often literally) forward. For years I hadn't thought about this except when I'd seen myself on television or heard myself interviewed on the radio. Now I was laughing so much I was hearing it repeated and magnified and I was becoming increasingly sensitive to it. With all the giggling in the room it was not the only thing giving me the sense of being returned to adolescence.

'How are you feeling?' Lotte asked me; and I said honestly, 'Surprisingly tired.'

It's the sort of flip comment that might usually raise a polite smile, an exhaled single-syllable chuckle of agreement. But here everyone laughed and then they wouldn't stop. At first I felt like I'd said something very clever, but as the honking, snorting cackles resounded around me I looked at the group – the woman in her bright yellow top with a huge M&M Smiley on it and another with a cap and glasses with bright frames – and felt that there was a touch of the circus about our little troupe.

I'd say I laugh quite often and that I make small jokes as ways to make connections with people. But here that felt like saying that you buy drinks to make friends – or that you distribute crack cocaine: every time I offered some lame witticism this lot were getting their fix. My out-sniff of a quiet laugh was picked up and used as material for more until the place had exploded. I worried then that I was actually the material, and it didn't make me feel funnier; it made me profoundly uncomfortable.

For the final activity of the morning, Lotte got us lying down, heads touching, bodies radiating out like the spokes of a wheel. She invited us to laugh with our eyes closed.

'But the laughing now is optional,' she said.

I am a good girl – give me rules and I will follow them. If we'd been told to laugh then, as in the other exercises, I would have done so. But since it had been offered, I took the option and didn't join in this laughter. Around me the room rang and shuddered with hoots and gurgles and snickers. I started to regret my decision not to take part, but once you've set yourself apart from laughter it's hard to join in, and even though I knew that no-one but Lotte could see that I wasn't participating, I felt self-conscious in my silence. With my eyes closed, and for the benefit of no-one but myself (and possibly Lotte) I adopted an amused – or perhaps bemused – smile. It was like being the only teetotaller at a party, or the only sane one at the asylum. Or like being in the corner of the playground surrounded by the sounds of jeering; the feeling that the joke is on you. It was a final reminder of the power of laughter, and the importance of using it wisely.

After the session, slightly unsettled by my experience, I had the chance to talk to the other women (Lotte said that more women come to her training, though men are starting). As conversation unfolded I was reminded of the brave painted smile of the clown, the town's fireworks going ahead even in the rain.

'I've had depression since I was young,' said Jenny (now sixty-two). 'I've had suicidal thoughts. And then I read about Laughter Yoga in a magazine and thought I'd like to try it. This is only the second day I've been doing it, but when I went home last night I realised that at last I was laughing not from here,' she pointed at her chest, 'but from my belly.'

Jools added that she knew the power of Laughter Yoga from having done a session with someone else. 'After a class you feel exhaustion, exhilaration; but that a weight's been lifted off you,' she said. She was a teacher of regular yoga who wanted to incorporate Lotte's techniques into her classes, which include seated yoga teaching for older people whom she thinks can particularly benefit from unconditional laughter.

H was another of the participants and told me about the 'serious bereavement' she had experienced and the support she'd had from Laughter Yoga. 'You've got to stop relying on others to make you laugh,' she said. 'That's what you learn from Laughter Yoga. It's better not to rely on jokes or other people's humour but instead just choose to laugh for no reason every day.

'When I was going through that bereavement, it was because we were laughing for no reason that I felt I could do it,' she explained. 'For nine years I've been doing Laughter Yoga most days. Of course I do lapse some days but I notice the effects when that happens.'

As I walked through the town to the station I learned a new way of listening to the people around me. I spotted the 'ha ha ha' of the men smoking outside one of the gay bars on Queen Street, the 'hee hee' of a mother with her child, the polite chuckle of a shopkeeper to a customer's pleasantry; I could sense the endorphins flowing. I thought about illness, about bereavement, about flying the flag on Blackpool Tower even when it was obscured by cloud and I knew that not everyone's laughter is because they're healthy and happy; but that we can all laugh because that is how we want to be.

Gratitude diary entry
my hoodie – its warmth and pillowing and seventeen years of service

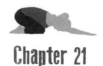

Chapter 21

The Mandala Yoga Ashram, Carmarthenshire

'Have no expectations'

There are only four trains a day from Shrewsbury to the station where you can get a taxi to the Mandala Yoga Ashram at Llanwrda. I was on the last of the day's trains, and its two carriages were emptying with every stop. The train carried people to what was billed as the 'Heart of Wales' but this felt like a marketing spin on 'Middle of Nowhere'. But if you're on a spiritual journey then getting to the middle of anything was to be applauded. And getting to nowhere was the perfect yogic journey.

Nevertheless, the sense of eeriness increased with each person who left the train. Night had fallen outside and my phone had run out of battery. From what seemed to me to have been cosy, Anglo-Saxon place names we had first stopped at (*Church Stretton, Broome, Hopton Heath*), we were now passing through settlements I had never heard of. I heard a fellow passenger asking whether we were stopping at one of the many stops whose name began with 'Llan'. He pronounced it with an English 'L' and the Welshman he was speaking to looked at him with genuine confusion. Other Welsh speakers around clarified in a chorus of throat-gargling. It didn't help to remember my Cornish lessons and see a cousin of the 'lan' I'd learned in another Celtic outpost; this was unknown country I couldn't even pronounce. I was starting to feel very alone.

The husky-toned yogini inside me said *that's because we* are *all alone.*

I pulled my rucksack closer to me on the seat as the train trundled on through the dark, occasionally escorted by the banshee calls of level-crossing sirens which had shut rural roads to make way for our coming. Wales indeed.

I was travelling to experience the 'karma yoga' offered in the form of meaningful work through the communal living of an ashram. It had sounded like an extremely cool thing to be doing when I'd mentioned it in emails to friends. But now I realised that I didn't exactly know what an ashram was. And I couldn't even use my phone to google it. In fact I wouldn't be able to use my phone to google it until I'd left, since I'd been informed with the message that confirmed my reservation for a night at the Mandala community that whatever the ashram was, it was not a place that had Wi-Fi.

I had been to one ashram before, on a gap-year visit to India twenty-five years earlier. I hadn't stayed the night, and the only thing I could remember about it was the spreading of liquid cow dung on the floor and the explanation of how it kept the place cool.

My reservation confirmation had also explained that my share of the Mandala Ashram's karma yoga could include cleaning of the common areas, so I was preparing for a day of cow dung spreading. I remembered the woman in the sari in 1990s India making beautiful swooshes across the floor as she layered the shit around our feet. I knew I would not be able to make nearly such a neat job of it.

The only other spiritual community I had stayed at was a monastery carved into the rock face halfway up a mountain in the Syrian desert. My lasting memory was of breakfasting on flatbreads, and olives from the monastery's recently planted trees. The olives were pea-sized, meaning that they were more like stones surrounded by a skin and bitter oily slime. On the assumption that spiritual community breakfasts might all be alike, I had this afternoon stuffed some salt and vinegar crisps into my rucksack.

The confirmation details and attached housekeeping information ('candles and incense are not to be burned') had also explained that the ashram has a rule of silence every night from 9pm. My train was due in at 8.53pm.

That the taxi (the 'tacsi'; we were in Wales now) was at the station at all started to rewrite the narrative I'd been constructing. That it was driven by a friendly guy called Ian who'd taken 'thousands' of people to the ashram before helped too.

'But there have been some,' he counted on the fingers of one hand, 'who I've dropped off and the next day had a call to come and take home.'

'Really? But why?'

He didn't answer and I thought of animal sacrifice and tantric sex and whistleblowing and started to panic.

'But you've got my phone number,' he joked, 'so you can always call if you want pizza.'

I asked what the local attitudes to the ashram were.

'When it opened I thought it was a cult,' he admitted. 'But I've learned more about it now. I know a driver locally who suffers from stress and depression who's been wondering whether he should go for a stay. No-one would know he was just down the road – and he could come home when he needs a shower.'

I disregarded the testimonial for the ashram as a place where taxi drivers could heal and skipped straight to a new nervousness: so, was this famously a place without showers? And I wondered where Ian's suspicion had come from.

He told me about the local economy. 'Round here it's mainly farming – some dairy but mainly sheep and some beef.' Maybe it was a tough crowd to sell a vegetarian lifestyle to. But who made up this 'crowd' anyway? As the headlights picked up swirling mist and high hedgerows, and the car swerved in the darkness around potholes and down lanes, I had seen not a single sign of habitation on our journey from the station. And I had no idea where I was.

None of us have any idea where we are, said that voice. It had taken on a ghoulish echo to match the wraiths outside.

'And I'll tell you another thing,' Ian said as we came to a passing place created in the narrow lane, 'just remember this passing place and in a little bit I'll tell you a story.' I duly noted it, and we drove on up the lane, round corners and on for many minutes in the darkness.

'So my story took place here,' said Ian. 'You've seen how far we came from that passing place, but look here,' he gestured out the window about ten metres from where he'd got my attention, 'there's another passing place.'

'There was a woman driving back from the ashram and we met just here. Someone had to reverse because this is so tight. She had ten metres to reverse to get to a passing place. Or I could go for half a mile backwards to that place we saw before. She absolutely refused to reverse even though it made sense for both of us. I waited and gestured but in the end I had to turn back half a mile. And she was coming from a stay at the ashram!'

It was a good reminder of the reality of karma yoga and the application of principles off the mat. Anyone can be tolerant and wise and peace-loving in Shavasana; this stay at the ashram was going to be my test of whether that could be sustained and deepened by living the principles, even if only for twenty-four hours. I hoped I'd do better than the driver who'd so enraged Ian.

Eventually we drove past a signpost for the ashram, and a gate, but even once we were through there was a long, unlit and twisting driveway. The bouncing headlights picked out a tall figure in a black coat whose silhouette showed Basil Rathbone features, standing at the side of the drive. I glanced at my watch; it was past 9pm: the man wouldn't speak to me even if I greeted him.

Ian must have seen something pass over my expression.

'Don't worry; you can call me,' he said again, half-joking still. 'And if we find bodies when we arrive then I promise I won't leave. I think that guy did have a knife.'

I looked at his face; Ian was enjoying himself.

Finally we pulled up at the house and Ian got out to help me wrestle the rucksack out of the boot. We confirmed the time he'd pick me up the next day.

'Do you need all of this stuff just for one night?' he asked. 'You could actually leave it in the car if not.'

My rucksack is a difficult child that everyone wants to mother somehow. But right now I wasn't letting anything familiar out of my sight.

As we negotiated I heard light footsteps and turned to see jolting torchlight approaching. This must be Maha Sattwa who had promised she would be waiting to greet me.

She spoke to me! Despite all the images of weird rites that had been swirling before my nervous gaze as I stared out at the mist on this journey, in fact the thing that had been bothering me most was how I was going to be welcomed to the ashram after 9pm when no-one was speaking. 'Silence until the group chanting session in the morning'. But Maha Sattwa spoke to me! She was a smiling, practical woman younger than me. She handed me a torch, checked that my journey had been OK, and led me past outbuildings and up a path to what my guttering torch showed through the mist to be the house where I'd be spending the night. She pushed open the door and took her shoes off to enter so I hurried to follow suit, though I was carrying a twenty-five kilogram rucksack on my back and my boots had zips. The rucksack made me unbalance, and I drew on all my core strength and skills of balance honed in my session with Prema to keep upright.

Once Maha Sattwa had shown me the door of my room, and told me that my roommate was called Samantha, she was off. And at that moment the battery in my torch died.

So I pushed open the door of the room, and found Samantha reading in her bed.

'Hi!' I said. She waved sheepishly back but since it was after 9pm of course she didn't talk to me. I was taken back to my days at boarding school. I felt like I'd been sent to Coventry.

I lurched my rucksack off my back and onto the bed, and the mattress echoed my sigh. All I had to do now was to – mindfully and unobtrusively – get myself into this bed.

But first I discovered there were no sheets on the bed. Perhaps Maha Sattwa had forgotten. I ran out after my guide and called into the chilly ink-blackness.

'Maha Sattwa! Maha Sattwa?' There was no response and I remembered the 9pm rule. Very quietly I returned to my room. Samantha had her face turned away when I entered.

Later I learned that I had been expected to bring my own sheets, but for now I made do with my old friend, the travelling Indian bedspread.

And there were other things to organise before I could get into this makeshift burrow. Given that I'd been travelling most of the day to get here, and that the next day I would be off again, I felt a pressing need to sort my devices.

My laptop had run out of battery en route so I had to plug it in. I tried to do it mindfully. Then I needed to set my alarm for tomorrow morning since I was decidedly travel-weary. To set an alarm I needed to plug in my dead phone too. With limited sockets, that meant unplugging the bedside light. All this was of course done very mindfully too, though perhaps not entirely silently.

And then there was my Kindle. On the long journey here I had also finished reading the paperback I'd brought. The Kindle needed a USB port to charge. The devices lined up like little gods on my bedside table altar and I was aware of the watchful gaze of Samantha, wrapped up in bed unspeakingly.

Now all I needed was to change into some nightwear. I knew which pocket of my rucksack those things were so with the minimum of noise to disturb Samantha's meditation/drishti, I unzipped the pocket. There was a loud crackling. Oh God! It was also in this pocket that I had squeezed the bag of salt and vinegar crisps. It is almost impossible to extract a bag of salt and vinegar crisps soundlessly from a rucksack pocket. But they had to be extracted. And it was *very* quiet here. I felt like I would be able to hear someone pull a bag of crisps from a rucksack a mile away.

Then I had to get out my toiletries bag. The idea pleased me because I knew that this was an ethically-sourced unbleached cotton drawstring bag containing a wooden toothbrush, a bottle of rosewater cleanser to be used with organic cotton pads to clean my face before putting on a cream made from ethically-extracted snail mucus (this is true; it had been a gift). But it was regrettably under a bundle of Balkan social enterprise handcrafts that rustled and crunched as I moved them.

I had a naughty thrill knowing that Samantha *couldn't* say anything for another ten hours, however much I annoyed her.

Samantha tapped on her bedside table and I looked up. She was doing the only thing she could in the circumstances – turning the light off. And the torch from Maha Sattwa would be no use to get me to the bathroom.

Luckily, in the case of small peripherals in the bag within my day bag I kept another torch. Proudly I burrowed into the bag and brought out another piece of equipment. I had believed that with my luggage for any eventuality I was going to manage life at the ashram just fine. Now I wasn't quite sure.

Thanks to my devices, I was woken by an alarm in time to go out for one of my morning walks. The ashram's grounds were extensive and it took me a while to work out the location of the gate through which we had entered last night. It was closed but when I saw it I found myself walking down there just to touch it. I reminded myself that this wasn't boarding school; I could leave when I wanted. I had Ian's number, and now I even had a working phone. It was interesting how my exploration of yoga had led me to exploring institutions – here and in prison and in Peterborough's places of worship. I hadn't known yoga would take me to places I would find so uncomfortable.

It was chilly out and I headed back to the house, thinking I could sit and read for a while before the chanting would begin. With my back now to the gate I could see several buildings set amid rambling paths. With a familiar rising panic I wondered which was mine; last night's mist, darkness and glancing torchlight had been entirely disorienting. I set off up the path that seemed most likely and came to a door which opened and led into a hall which I knew immediately was not the space where I had wobbled on one leg last night, trying to take off my boots.

I tried another path but knew before I even reached the building that this wasn't right. I wandered round in this fashion, past the ashram's car workshop, the compost heaps, the vegetable patch and the labyrinth meditation space (ha! no need for that if you have the sense of direction that I do) for some time before finding topography which seemed familiar. It was the right hallway! Going into my room and finding Samantha there felt like being reunited with an old friend.

The danger of life on an ashram is that husky voice that had piped up repeatedly over the last twelve hours – you start to take everything metaphorically.

I sat silently on my bed reading through some of the leaflets I'd found here about the ashram. Ian had been right to be wary about the showers – the information explained that there was no mains water so we were warned that at certain times when there were lots of people staying there can be a drain on the tanks. And for mobile phones and computers the leaflet said briefly, 'keep them switched off'. I ruefully looked up at my little illuminated display of technology. The divine light in me salutes…

Shortly before the morning chant was due to start I left the house and walked down to the hall. An early morning yoga class was still in session. Through the French windows I could see the hall was full of bodies undulating in Cat-Cow backbends like a field of silent Friesians.

A cluster of us waited outside while their asanas came to an end and the class filed out and we took their places. There were bolsters and blankets available and each of the dozen or so of us here huddled in our spaces. I had been thinking of this morning communal chanting like the only morning religious observance I'd attended before – the dawn service for Easter morning in the village where I'd grown up. I'd expected a service of celebration – *Christ is risen; he is risen indeed! And here's a chocolate.* But the straggling people taking their places here, with our bed-messy hair and our outlandish clothes, looked like a crowd in search of refuge, not of rejoicing. Around the room the empty stomachs were anticipating breakfast. As we settled there was a sound as of wood pigeons or whale song.

The 'swami' entered – a man of middle age in a peach-coloured jumper and apricot shawl. It was more Marks and Spencer than I'd imagined a spiritual leader to be. I remembered the gnomic advice on the ashram's website within the tab about coming to stay and the section headed 'What to Expect' which read simply:

Have no expectations.

I was later to learn that Swamiji, to use his honorific title, is from Romford.

I found the chanting more complicated than I'd anticipated. There was the melody to master, but at the same time there were words in what I guessed was Sanskrit. I don't like singing something when I don't know what it means so I tried to follow not only in Sanskrit but also in the English translation, which we had printed on the bottom half of the page.

I was pleased when it was over and we were allowed to go to breakfast. Even if there were only tiny olives to break our bodies' fast, this was, more importantly, the moment when we could rectify the conversation deprivation we had put ourselves through.

It was better than olives – it was surprisingly delicious turmeric and black pepper porridge. Carrying it steaming fragrantly from my bowl I headed for Samantha, to apologise for last night's crisp packet.

She smiled at me when I sat next to her.

'Hey roomie,' she said. She smiled.

Have no expectations.

'It's so… so nice to hear you talk,' I said. 'It was really weird last night…'

'Yeah, I know,' she giggled.

Giggled!

Really, human relationships were a lot better when you didn't just communicate by rapping on your bedside table or by rattling your crisp packets.

Our chat was interrupted by a bell. One of the ashram residents sitting near us explained that was to say there was more porridge left. A porridge bell?

I felt a Pavlovian reaction building. Over the day I heard more echoes of boarding school as the bells multiplied. Bells to tell you when to do something; bells to tell you that soon you'd have to stop doing something. Years of training as a conscientious, prize-winning boarding school pupil meant that my instinct was to jump each time I heard one, and wonder what I was late for now.

The next one, we were informed, meant that karma yoga was to start. But Samantha and I were told first to report to the operations manager's office. I felt cheated – I wanted to get going with spreading dung on the floor, or with whatever task I had been allocated.

Nevertheless, we went obediently to Nick's office. He looked up from his computer as we entered and carefully took off his watch when he started talking to us, and lay it down on the desk. I wasn't sure if this was a symbol of removing himself from petty time commitments, or whether it was so he could anchor himself better to them by more easily seeing when our allotted time had come to an end. Maybe the watch just didn't feel comfortable.

He started with an explanation of the ashram and his role. Being operations manager for an ashram seemed contradictory somehow – like being the organiser of an anarchists' conference. But he talked about how he saw his contribution to the mission of the organisation, which he described as being 'a place for seekers'. 'It's a place for the big questions that we all ask when we're children, and then we stop asking them, or people don't allow us to ask them as we get older.'

It was also, he explained, a place for exploring the boundaries between work and life, for reflecting on how we integrate our values in our work. Whatever we were given to do, I prepared to take it as a case study. The voice inside me with a penchant for parable and metaphor started clearing its throat.

'I bet I'm on toilet cleaning,' I said to Samantha on the way out of the office. In a strange way I relished the idea – the humility it would require, the earthiness of it… We went to check the noticeboard; Samantha was on toilet cleaning. I was given the task of cleaning out the catering fridge.

I was bizarrely disappointed. I didn't think you'd catch Gandhi cleaning out a fridge. This was surely for the gentrified yogini. And I found fridges frustrating to clean – something about their surface which meant that stray drops from your cloth stayed there and you got none of the satisfaction you could get with a damp rag on a dusty table, for example; water pooled.

But of course I was here to learn the philosophy of work, and by God and by Krishna, if my allotted task was to clean a fridge then I would do it.

I set to, pulling out the many glass shelves and salad hoppers and piling them on the work surface behind me. It was a tight space to work, being the pantry off the kitchen, but there were vegetable racks tangy with onions, and sacks of lentils and brown rice and spice drawers gave off an exotic woody scent. I inhaled with an *ujjayi* breath and noted how mindful I was being.

Through the doorway, another ashram guest was preparing lunch for us all. Mina and I exchanged snatches of conversation in between our tasks. She had been here many times before and nodded approvingly at my work.

'Tony is the chef here during the week. He'll be so pleased to have a new fridge,' she said, and I beamed, reflecting on my motivation for doing work and my pleasure in pleasing others.

Systematically I went through the food in the fridge, identifying anything that needed to be thrown away, and swabbing at the turmeric stains I found. Tony was going to be so happy with this nice job.

When a bell rang for a (caffeine-free) tea break Samantha and I found each other again. I asked her how the work was going. She said she'd finished the toilets and had been told to mop the floor of the hallway where everyone took their shoes off.

'But one part of it has to be constantly redone because people keep coming in,' she grumbled. I was feeling so karmic and yogic about the nature of work that I smiled wisely at this. I knew the value of work – the pleasure that work could be in itself, unrelated to whether it needs to be redone. I mentioned the blowing up of the bridge on the River Kwai by the British colonel who had used its construction as the only way to stay sane. We nodded sagely, like our tea. I was proud of my work ethic.

'I think the floor mopping must be a job that's quite frequently done because other than the route that people walked through it didn't really need doing,' Samantha said. 'But I found some bits that hadn't been done in a while.' Newly reflective about our work, we shared notes on how satisfying that was, and how I'd had the same experience finding bits of gunge in the fridge, and taking pleasure in sorting out bits that other people had missed.

I became less proud of my work ethic: this didn't sound like karma yoga but an ego trip.

Back at work in the pantry, while at the stove Mina stirred the simmering leeks she was preparing for our proper Welsh lunch, she and I chatted some more. She asked me about my journey here, and my yoga adventures. I had just started telling her some of my highlights when from behind me came a crash followed by a smash, a splintering and a smithereen. Adrenaline lurched in me and I turned to see the broken remains of the tower of shelves and trays that I'd piled up as I'd taken them from the fridge. The damage was spectacular because the trays had shattered into fierce crystals, like windscreen glass after a car crash.

My cheeks flamed with shame and my eyes pricked with embarrassed and embarrassing tears.

'Oh my…' said Mina, and I knew she was thinking of Tony.

'I'm so sorry,' I said inadequately.

'I'm going to get Nick,' she said.

By the time they came back I had started picking glass out of the vegetable rack and sweeping at the crunchy glittering floor.

I guessed Nick was angry.

'I'm sorry,' I said again.

'Don't worry,' he attempted to reassure me. 'But how did it happen?' I couldn't explain. I'd not been mindful enough perhaps, with the tower I'd created on the side. Or perhaps it was just bad luck.

'I'll buy replacement shelves,' I promised but Nick shook his head.

'No-one is buying any replacements,' he said illogically, and left the room.

Why wouldn't he let me pay for the damage I'd caused? That could at least make up for what I'd done.

Ah! Just because of that, I realised. This was what it meant to be operations manager of an ashram; to think not only about balancing the budget line for refrigerators, but to balance the karma yoga needs of the community's members. And I was not going to be allowed to buy my way out of this bit of poor workmanship.

So I set to, trying to make it up with hard work. I pulled out all the sacks and the storage units from the pantry so as to sweep up the glass crumbs from every corner. While I was there I rubbed at sticky patches, cleaned up stains, put the onions back in orderly rows. And I tried to draw some conclusions. What had caused the crash? Had I not been careful enough? I'd been cold and tired, and thoughtless? I'd been talking to Mina.

A woman came into the kitchen and saw the devastation and my efforts at reconstruction.

'Wow, what happened?' she asked.

I told her. 'And I'm trying to learn some profound lesson from it,' I said ruefully as my dustpan squawked on the floor tiles over the glass gravel.

She shrugged. 'You just have to accept things,' she said, and turned away to begin vegetable peeling.

Did I? Could I just accept that in this case a chance current of air had shifted the balance of the stack of refrigerator trays?

Mina said helpfully that breaking things is good luck.

'And we were talking about your yoga journey when it happened,' so you know it's a blessing on you really.

Mina was being kind. But I was struggling with something that couldn't be made better with cute superstition. I'd come here to think about work and ethics and motivation and values in practice. I felt I was on the verge of learning something significant.

The pantry had been put back together, and the fridge was clean and restocked with everything except its two wrecked shelves.

'Mina, do you have some other job I could help you with?' I asked.

'Well, there's a roasting pan here with baked-on grease you could scour out?' she offered.

'No problem,' I said with relief.

'You're a very kind person, Elizabeth.'

I answered without even thinking, 'No, I'm just a very guilty person.'

As I rubbed and scrubbed at the stubborn grease on the roasting pan, I thought about this ready comment I'd made. I thought about the times I'd tried to do good work (and Good Works). And although I wasn't in the habit of destroying refrigerator shelving, I so often had things I felt guilty about. My work ethic felt as shattered as the poor old fridge.

But it usually served me so well. I knew what I had achieved – for myself and for others – from my hard work. I knew that even looking for the gunge that other people had left behind had led to me making small changes for the better in the world, and not just its pantries. But the guilt, the expectations I had of myself; were they a force for good in my life, or even in the lives of others?

Have no expectations.

A bell rang and I jumped again.

Could you just allow the bell to be a bell? my inner yogi asked me. No obligations, no expectations?

I could try.

But before I left the ashram, I noted down the model number of the fridge. When I got home I found a website that offered Beko spare parts and paid for replacement shelves to be delivered to Wales. Because guilt is powerful – and sometimes it pushes you to do things that make the world a slightly better place.

Gratitude diary entry
the towel I had carried with me for my travels, a present from a Kosovan friend and a bit of familiarity when I wake up in unfamiliar surroundings

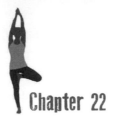

Chapter 22

In My End Is My Beginning –
Yin Yoga in Newquay

'You sure have a lot of wind beneath your wings'

It's less than twenty-four miles from Port Isaac to Newquay. By car it takes about forty-five minutes. By public transport it's two and a half hours, and three buses. The buses will get me there just a little faster than if I took the centuries-old Cornish sea route and rowed there by pilot gig.

But bus travel is one of the charms of my Cornish life. It might be that I only take the buses when I have time enough to enjoy their eccentricities, but there is an enforced leisure to the culture of the Duchy's buses which is rivalled only by the life of upper-middle-class women in Victorian England. Time does not waste you – here you devise ever more elaborate ways to waste it. This is the land of I-spy, of numberplate bingo, of looking out to be the first to spot the sea in order to earn sixpence (even the currency is that of those Victorian women). Time stops being something you wrestle panting to the ground, or a winged creature at your back, its breath hot on your neck. Time doesn't run through your fingers like spilt milk, here it thickens and clots like cream, becomes spreadable; something that tops even jam.

This leisurely 'yin' approach to travel was probably the most appropriate way to get to my destination today – Oceanflow Studio – avoiding frenetic Bikram motorways. And I came well-equipped for my long journey with an audio book (I had no travelling companion for I-spy). I was listening to the 1,700-year-old wisdom of the *Yoga Sutras of Patanjali* as the first of my buses trundled through the tight Cornish lanes bound with dry-stone walls, fringed with valerian and studded with beach asters:

> Undisturbed calmness of mind is attained by cultivating friendliness toward the happy, compassion for the unhappy, delight in the virtuous, and indifference toward the wicked.

> For those who have an intense urge for Spirit and wisdom, it sits near them, waiting.

> Sloth is the great enemy – the inspirer of cowardice, irresolution, self-pitying grief, and trivial, hairsplitting doubts.

> The strident vibrations of selfishness, lust and hate are to be stilled by meditation.

When travelling I listen to books rather than reading them because if I try reading while I'm on the move I get motion sickness right away. But audio books have another benefit, which is that they free your eyes. As Patanjali's sutras flowed from my earphones I could focus on hedgerows and seascapes but also on the people around me. It was a busy bus – the transport for kids at the secondary school who live in the surrounding villages. And today each of the teenagers was dressed in shorts and sweatshirt, with the nervy expectation that precedes Sports Day. The bus driver asked them about it and gave avuncular advice about winning. He was a law unto himself, self-appointed mayor of a traditional but fair little community on the move, demanding of the lads that they give up their seats for older or female passengers, stopping briefly without explanation at Barnecutt's to jump out and buy a pasty just before we reached the depot, and implementing his own brand of moral code when I helped out a walker who boarded with only a twenty-pound note to pay with.

The driver had said he couldn't accept the note and I'd seen the sudden panic on the walker's face. I knew the next bus wouldn't be for two hours and I remembered, too, a day when I had been on this bus on the way to the train station, hurrying for an important connection to get up to London. The same thing had happened to me – my proffered twenty-pound note, a driver refusing it, and the threat that without that ticket, without that bus, I would miss that train and my appointment in London. I had been saved then by an older woman sitting in one of the 'reserved for passengers who find it hard to stand' seats.

'You don't know me, but I know you,' she'd said. She was the next-door neighbour of a friend of mine, and she handed over the four-pound fare for me. I had tried paying her back at the time, rifling in my purse and desperately offering her postage stamps in compensation. She'd smiled and refused, and now – perhaps three years later – I found my chance to pay it back. Perhaps I could settle my debt to Trish in Liverpool at the same time.

So as the walker's face fell and he contemplated two hours' waiting at the bus stop, two hours of daylight lost, two hours of stumbling along roads at dusk, and delay in arrival at wherever he was to be staying that night, I told him I'd pay his fare.

He didn't travel as far as I did and when I was preparing to get off the bus after he'd left, the driver called me up to the front to 'settle up'. I went up to the little Perspex window with a frown.

'I'm not charging you for this journey,' he said, and with a clink of coins he pressed the pneumatic button to open the doors for me, like a junior St Peter.

When the next bus arrived, and now we were away from the school-run timetable, it was eerily empty. But there was still plenty to look at – this vehicle came together with Cornish lessons. Like the bus gannin' along the Scotswood Road in Newcastle this local transport company was taking a similar opportunity to celebrate and educate while they built their brand loyalty and local pride. An annotated illustration taught me how to say in Cornish 'a man taking a selfie' (*den owth omskeusa*), along with the rather more useful 'bus' (*kyttrin*), 'driver' (*lewyer*) and 'return please' (*mos ha dos mar pleg*).

Almost the only other passengers were a mother and her skinny, reluctant-looking teenage son. I wondered what they were doing out during school hours. Home education? Medical appointment? At the next stop the mum got off and kissed the lad goodbye. A few stops later we arrived at the school bus stop and the woman driving the bus called out the school's name. Encouragingly, she added to the teenager, 'This is for you then sweetheart. Have a good day!' I felt I'd met the mayor, or perhaps the social worker, of another small and temporary community.

My final bus of the journey was a new model, even equipped with USB charging facilities. It had more passengers than the last one, so I had new entertainment. I didn't feel bad about listening in to their conversations as I'd learned from my first bus journeys in Cornwall that what you said here was considered public property – like the

CCTV recordings on public transport which are then beamed onto the screens as you're travelling. On an early bus journey I had been discussing my shopping chores in Wadebridge with my travelling companion. I was wondering where I could get shoes reheeled and the young guy in front of us had turned round, just as if he'd been asked. He'd given us careful and accurate directions to the cobbler's shop I needed. Since then I'd refrained from any more personal conversations on First Kernow transport.

I didn't interrupt others but I did listen in as the young couple in front of me planned their day in Newquay. The guy had been before and was giving the benefit of his experience to his girlfriend. His summary was simple: 'The town is shit but the beaches are nice.'

As an introduction it seemed fair as I made my way down the main shopping street past hair braiders, dream-catchers and the Oldest Cornish Pasty Maker in the World. This was a town flooded by the sea and by the fruits of the sea. It milled with tourists drawn by the spectacular beaches, and it dripped with what had come out of the ocean. Today that was less likely to be a fisherman's catch, and more often the damp wetsuits which hung drying from balconies like slick mackerel would have done a century ago.

A population swollen and distended by such visitors is not always a comfortable experience for the host community, and Newquay's visitors have a reputation for bad behaviour, but I saw only indulgence, tolerance and hospitality for these blow-ins. It was a hot day and it was the kind of place where bowls of water were left outside people's gates for passing dogs.

Beyond the main shops, I carried on past a small informal community hub that had grown up at a crossroads – the adult education centre, and halls for the WI and the Salvation Army (and a funeral director). I passed houses with brilliant names like Sea La Vie and Salty Towers.

But I was looking for a place called Gwelva Lowenek. The little Cornish I'd learned on my short course (as well, of course, from the bus company's tuition) helped me to understand the second word, which shared a root with the Cornish girl's name, Lowena. It means 'happy' and the whole name meant 'happy viewpoint', which seemed a perfect location for a yoga studio.

As I got closer to where I thought it should be, I saw a woman whom I was pretty sure was heading to yoga class. It might have been her aura and my new sensitivities to psychic energy. But it was probably the large roll she was carrying under her arm... Unless you mistake a bazooka gun, yoga practitioners are pretty easy to identify. I guess that double-bass players must have a similar way of recognising one another on their way to practice.

When we got to Oceanflow it turned out to be a modest terraced house given yogic touches by some careful design. Outside, a wooden plinth bore the *om* sign and a sun-bleached Adirondack chair tilted back to catch the sun, dappled by agapanthus plants.

The studio is owned by a couple whose names sound like a yoga enterprise's perfect combination of knowledge and physical challenge. The business belonging to Jen and Stretch (he's tall) has been voted 'best yoga studio in Cornwall' three years in a row.

There was a small reception where I asked about my travelling companion, the unyogic rucksack. The rucksack had been a good friend to me: a rock to lean on – as well as a boulder to carry around Britain. I had dozed on it, sat on it, eaten lunch off it – and of course been grateful for the things I carried in it. Leaning my head on it on the seat next to me on bus and train journeys or as I waited at stations, I had learned its anatomy, and how to find its softest parts; nuzzling it I knew where I'd find familiar patches of sweat and dust and washing powder.

But it was a terrible liability when I arrived at a yoga studio. For a start, it marked me out as passing through: it begged questions. It required storage, and on its way through crowded or confined spaces it knocked pictures off walls and scuffed paintwork. I found myself spending much of my time explaining or apologising for it, like one might do for an unruly child. People will put out bowls of water for passing dogs but they tend to be much less welcoming of passing rucksacks.

At Oceanflow they were unbothered by it and Holly, the yoga teacher for my yin class, took us both up to the changing room. It was a small, pretty space with curtains and screens that made it more boudoir than locker room. I put my smaller bag on one of the shelves. The shelf above it sprouted green leaves – a bundle of kale left there as if the room might offer material for every possible mind-body-spirit trend.

I commented on the kale to the teacher and she parted the bundle to show me that it had been left there together with a pineapple-shaped frame with a drawing and message on it – both gifts for her from one of her students after Holly had used the image of a pineapple in a previous class, as a meditation on being 'sweet and upright'. I realised I had come across my third community leader of the day.

While we were talking I had tried to stash my own sweet upright in an unobtrusive corner. The rucksack was more potato than pineapple and in that space it stood out like a hitchhiker's sore thumb. I felt it needed explanation...

'I'm doing quite a lot of travelling...' I said lamely, and then defensively named a random selection of the distant places I'd covered on the journey, to show that I was serious. It was a litany I was getting used to reciting, and people's reactions were usually something between pity and awe. Holly just said:

'You sure have a lot of wind beneath your wings.'

It was an empowering image: a lifted aeroplane; a soaring bird, and as I walked away from the rucksack and towards class with her, I felt effortless and light. As I listened more to her through the class I also learned it was a very yin thing to say – a focus on the support you have rather than on the effort you make.

Then we opened the door to the studio space where the world suddenly opened out. You didn't have to do Lion pose for your jaw to drop: the room looked out over the length of Fistral Bay where the legendary surf was drawing in and out with a reassuring ujjayi breath.

This coast was the first place I had ever done yoga without an instructor or video. It had taken me two years of regular practice before I felt bold enough to attempt even a Sun Salutation without someone calling out the breaths (the 'rules'). But it had been when walking beside this seascape and alone one morning on a clifftop that I'd had the urge to try – a quick, self-conscious Sun Salutation – with this ocean as my teacher.

It felt like an active participant in the session here today, with its breathing and its great chest-opening expanse. When Holly told us 'you may like to close your eyes' I didn't want to – I wanted to take every possible chance to gorge on the sight.

It seemed like a wonderful metaphor for us to focus on, too. Holly talked about exploring our limits during the session, and beyond; working out whether what we perceive as limits are set by our bodies or our minds. I considered her question about whether I could transcend those boundaries, while gazing out over the limits of the land.

There were seven other women in the class (I found the one with the tattoos and the coloured hair) and a gentle energy of strong bodies at rest. Holly began the session inviting us to sit with our feet together and our knees out. It's exactly what I'd been asked to do the previous day in my smear test which wasn't a great start, but she kept me focused. She talked us through imagining ourselves climbing the stairs to the studio, walking inside and shutting the door, leaving outside any anxieties or concerns. It was a simple trick, but it worked, and I forgot the doctor's appointment. She showed us how to hold our hands in *hridaya* mudra, forefinger coiled into the crook between it and thumb, and middle and ring fingers touched to thumb. She explained it was a position for freeing up blockages to your heart centre. A book I read later suggested trying this mudra during a disagreement in order to boost your compassion.

Today we were concentrating on the heart space because Holly explained that according to Chinese medicine the heart and the small intestine are the organs to focus on from 21 June and into August. She was wearing a heart necklace (I noted she had wisely chosen that design rather than a small intestine) and invited us as we started the day's practice to think about this part of our body and give it a colour and a texture. She suggested green or pink or gold, but the happiest colour and texture I could think of at that moment was washed blue denim – the colour of the sea we were gazing at, but also of the bolsters we'd each been given, for straddling in Hero pose, and for leaning back against.

The yin approach in this class was different from all the yoga I'd done before, focused on a small number of poses, each held for between three and five minutes. The theory was that this worked not the muscles but the connective tissues – 'fascia', tendons and ligaments. Everyone I've asked is at great pains to explain fascia to me but it always ends up grossing me out. My image of a muscle is of a spindle shape, a corn on the cob. So when people talk about the 'fascia' encasing our muscles the image I have in my mind is of the membrane you have to peel off between the corn and the leaves. And then I imagine it in my own body and I feel queasy again.

The yin approach sees itself as different from the more 'yang' exertions of vinyasa flow. It's described as 'innercise as well as exercise'. Holly reminded us about the body's reactions to pain – the release of adrenaline and cortisol, the tensing of muscles, the increase of heart rate and blood pressure. Put like that, it seemed obvious that pain was something that we wouldn't want to inflict on our bodies. She invited us to explore the difference between pain and tingling or other sensations, and to place our practice at the best point.

Yin yoga's slow approach means that in an hour's class we did perhaps just six poses, held for five minutes each side. We started with a 'banana bend', our feet moving to the bottom right-hand corner of the mat while our hands went up to the top right-hand corner; we held a simple twist lying down with our knees over one side as we looked out over the other side; we sat in a modified Hero pose, our feet together and knees bent out to the side as we lent back against the bolster, our arms cradling our heads 'as if you're watching the clouds go by,' said Holly.

Which sounded very Huck Finn to start with, but as the seconds and minutes mounted, the discomfort built. I felt the impact of all my recent travelling – the overnight buses, the carried burdens, the uncomfortable seats, the lack of sleep. I wished I'd organised my time differently. I wished I was more flexible. I had thought that I was able to do more. Holly had warned us to let go of judgements of what we were doing, but I had felt myself tense at that. I never want to let go of those; I wanted to keep my critical faculties. Maybe it was one thing I did share with Laurette of PraiseMoves, but I wasn't ready yet to leave that space for other people's ideas to be inserted while I was looking elsewhere; or for brain and heart to be so disassociated.

At length we were able to move on to another side or another pose. The stamina needed for the practice reminded me of shifting a heavy shoulder bag while you're travelling – when you move it onto the other shoulder you first get a delicious feeling of ease on the side you'd just been stretching, but before you've walked much further, the strain begins to tell on the other side...

Holly took our minds off it with a quiet soundtrack of Indian and other music, against which she gave gentle readings and commentary on the theme for the day. This was 'blessings', and the practices of gratitude and compassion that come from them. Her voice was soft with an accent somewhere between the USA, where she was born, and Canada and Sweden, where she lived before coming to Cornwall. She used excerpts from *The Gentle Art of Blessing* and about the process of blessing as a gentle demonstration of well-wishing to others or yourself. She said she had been trying a practice of blessing her day before she gets up in the morning. Later I talked to her about the similarities of this with my gratitude diary habit.

Holly's explanations and examples of blessing were practical – yoga for living real life, for dealing with 'the days when the kids are screaming, when you're late for work and there's yet another set of temporary roadworks; when there are so many people in front of you in the queue in Sainsbury's'. How, she asked, can we show compassion in these circumstances? She started from a very Cornish point of departure, suggested being grateful for the fact that people were here on what she called *vacation*.

At the end of the session we moved into Shavasana, and Holly said she would come round with an eye mask for each of us. She asked us to put a hand on our stomach if for some reason we didn't want the eye mask to be placed. It was like the subtle sign I'd been taught to give as a child in church if you were not confirmed, so as to receive a blessing at the altar rail rather than communion. It reminded me, too, of the discreet etiquette of tea-drinking in Kosovo where I'd learned to place a spoon over the top of my teaglass, with the bowl of the spoon convex, to signify that I didn't want more. My favourite kind of rituals lie somewhere between religion and a tea party.

An eye mask sounded luxurious so I kept my hands away from my stomach. When Holly came to me she placed an aromatic mask on my eyes, and her hands on my shoulders with gentle downward pressure. It realigned me with a feeling of release, as if I'd just taken off a pair of cramping shoes that my whole body had been compensating for. Afterwards, when I spoke to her about this, she said that she spoke a blessing over each person as she did it.

My Shavasana was deep and restorative. I remembered a description I'd read by columnist Jim Duffy:

> It's not like post-coital emotion. It's not like warming down after a 10K run. ... It feels like I would want to feel on the hour of my deathbed. Very calm. Very confident. Just me and my being.

That was it.

Sitting up gently from Shavasana, each of us found a small glittery heart sticker laid at the front of our mats. Holly has a touch of the tooth fairy about her.

It was a good prompt to think of all the gifts that I'd found on my mat and everything that yoga had brought me. I was bendier now than when I'd creaked and snapped like driftwood with the ladies in my first Port Isaac yoga class. But I'd also expanded my understanding of what yoga could mean. I'd learned that it could be hot, airborne, soft or stony. It could mean a giggle, a resonating sound, the shudder of a shaking muscle held in an awkward Kundalini pose, or the wobble of a gentle swell under my paddleboard; it could be a hand in an elegant stretch for Lululemon perfection, or shakily offering help and companionship during life-limiting conditions or life sentences. It might be the hand of a schoolchild, or your own hand re-experienced in a mudra; it may not even be a hand, but a paw. It's something you do in your own body and your own mind, that somehow connects you to the minds and bodies of those around you.

I gave thanks for all those who had taken me on this journey. And then I did what the best yoga prepares you for: I rolled up my mat and walked out – tall – into the world.

Gratitude diary entry
waking to the sound of the sea

Glossary

Asana – a pose held within yoga

Drishti – a focused gaze

Iyengar – B K S Iyengar (1918–2014) was the founder of a school of yoga particularly concentrating on the details and alignment in holding asanas

Kundalini – refers to energy said to be coiled at the base of the spine. A Kundalini approach to yoga focuses on movements and breathing designed to awaken this energy

Namaste – a greeting. It is often translated as meaning 'the divine light in me salutes the divine light in you'

Nidra – the Sanskrit word for 'sleep'

Om – considered to be 'the primordial sound', and a particularly resonant syllable which is often chanted to begin and/or end a yoga or meditation session

Prana – the breath, energy or life force

Pranayama – the regulation of the breath

Shavasana – literally means 'corpse pose' and is usually held at the end of a yoga session, lying flat on your back with palms upward and body relaxed

Trikonasana – Triangle pose; legs wide and one hand on the ground with the other reaching upwards

Ujjayi – a kind of breathing with a constriction in the throat leading to a rasping sound, sometimes called 'ocean breath', which helps with focusing on the breath

Vinyasa – a Sanskrit term for linking postures in a flowing movement

Yama –   a form of 'restraint' or discipline for 'right living'

Yogini –   female practitioner of yoga

Zafu –   a small round, densely stuffed cushion used for sitting on for meditation

Directory

Stand-Up Paddleboard Yoga in Nottingham – **f** SUP Yoga & Fitness UK

Brimham Rocks – **w** nationaltrust.org.uk/brimham-rocks

Lululemon, Edinburgh – **w** info.lululemon.co.uk/stores/gb/ edinburgh/edinburgh-store/events/hair-of-the-downward-dog

Jack Irvine, Edinburgh – **w** shanticollective.co.uk/our-teachers

Hot Yoga, Brighton – **w** yogahaven.co.uk/brighton-hove/yoga

Prison Phoenix Trust – **w** theppt.org.uk

Chris Holt – **w** yogawithchris.co.uk

OURMALA – **w** ourmala.com

Carolyn Fuest – **w** breathefreely.co.uk

Upala-haven Yoga, West Kilbride – **f** Upala-haven Yoga

The Fitness Hangout, Godalming – **w** thefitnesshangout.co.uk

DogaMahny ™ – **w** dogamahny.com

PraiseMoves – **w** praisemoves.com

The Inner Temple, Cirencester – **w** inner-temple.com

Sound Bath, The Vault, Wallsend – **w** the-vault.org/
regular-groups.html

The Iyengar Institute, Maida Vale – **w** iymv.org

Yoga Nidra with Uma Dinsmore-Tuli – **w** yoganidranetwork.org/
users/uma

Kalyani Yoga – **w** kalyaniyoga.co.uk

Brahma Kumaris – **w** brahmakumaris.org

Rosemary Prema Bennett, Liverpool – **w** premayoga.co.uk

Laughter Yoga – **w** lottemikkelsen.com

The Mandala Yoga Ashram – **w** mandalayogaashram.co.uk

Oceanflow Yoga, Newquay – **w** oceanflowyoga.co.uk

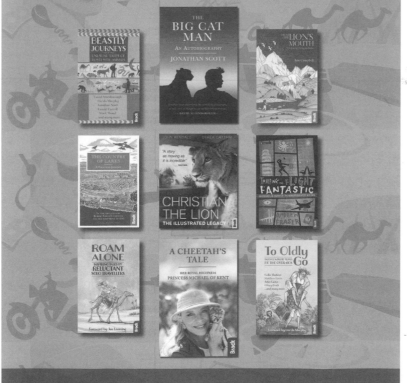